Dual Diagnosis.
Practice in Context

Dual Diagnosis: Practice in Context

Edited by

Dr Peter Phillips
(City University London)

Dr Olive McKeown
(St George's University, London)

and

Tom Sandford
(Royal College of Nursing, London)

WILEY-BLACKWELL

A John Wiley & Sons, Ltd., Publication

This edition first published 2010
© 2010 Blackwell Publishing Ltd

Blackwell Publishing was acquired by John Wiley & Sons in February 2007. Blackwell's publishing programme has been merged with Wiley's global Scientific, Technical, and Medical business to form Wiley-Blackwell.

Registered office
John Wiley & Sons Ltd, The Atrium, Southern Gate, Chichester, West Sussex, PO19 8SQ, United Kingdom

Editorial offices
9600 Garsington Road, Oxford, OX4 2DQ, United Kingdom
2121 State Avenue, Ames, Iowa 50014-8300, USA

For details of our global editorial offices, for customer services and for information about how to apply for permission to reuse the copyright material in this book please see our website at www.wiley.com/wiley-blackwell.

The right of the author to be identified as the author of this work has been asserted in accordance with the Copyright, Designs and Patents Act 1988.

Library of Congress Cataloging-in-Publication Data

Dual diagnosis : practice in context / edited by Peter Phillips, Olive McKeown, Tom Sandford.
    p. ; cm.
  Includes bibliographical references and index.
  ISBN 978-1-4051-8009-2 (pbk. : alk. paper) 1. Dual diagnosis. I. Phillips, Peter, 1968- II. McKeown, Olive. III. Sandford, Tom.
  [DNLM: 1. Diagnosis, Dual (Psychiatry) 2. Mental Disorders – complications. 3. Substance-Related Disorders – complications. WM 270 D8127 2010]
  RC564.68.D794 2010
  362.29 – dc22

                                                                                2009020246

A catalogue record for this book is available from the British Library.

Set in 10/12.5pt Palatino by Laserwords Private Limited, Chennai, India

1   2010

Contents

Contributors

Editors

Peter Phillips PhD, MSc, RMN, PGCAP, FHEA
Peter is senior lecturer in substance use and addiction in the School of Community & Health Sciences at City University London, and honorary lecturer in the Department of Mental Health Sciences at University College London Medical School. Peter trained as a mental health nurse in Leeds and after qualifying, worked in the Alcohol Unit at the Maudsley Hospital (London), and later in other specialist mental health, drug and alcohol and harm reduction services in London. He worked as a dual diagnosis nurse specialist in East London Harm Reduction Services, prior to obtaining a research fellowship at University College London Medical School in 1998, where he completed his PhD on the motivations for substance use in people with severe and enduring mental illnesses. In 2003, Peter received a Band Trust scholarship to investigate dual diagnosis in Northern India. During his time at University College London, Peter maintained a clinical link with Camden & Islington Mental Health Trust, where he implemented and later evaluated interventions to reduce drug-related deaths. Peter's research interests include folk pharmacology, dual diagnosis, harm reduction, and heroin overdose prevention strategies. Peter is a member of the International Advisory Board of Mental Health and Substance Use: dual diagnosis.

Olive McKeown PhD, MSc, Dip N, CELTT, Cert Obst, RMN, RGN
Olive is the lead tutor for problem-based learning (PBL) for the 4-year fast-track undergraduate medical programme at George's Medical School in SW London. She is also a visiting lecturer at the University of Greenwich contributing to substance misuse, dual diagnosis and adolescent mental health courses. Olive trained as an adult nurse in Lewisham and Guy's and undertook mental health nursing at the Bethlem Royal and Maudsley hospitals. She has worked in general medicine and surgery, specialist and

generic mental health, child and adolescent and drug and alcohol services. Subsequently, she worked as a lecturer practitioner within an acute in-patient service at Oxleas NHS Trust in SE London, where she began to develop a strong interest in dual diagnosis, prior to taking up a post as senior lecturer in substance misuse and mental health at the University of Greenwich in 1998. In 2004, Olive completed her PhD in mental health nursing, focusing on dual diagnosis within acute mental health settings. Olive's research and teaching interests include dual diagnosis, drug and alcohol use in young people, physical health and well-being in mental health patients as well as group dynamics within PBL groups and PBL as a means of curriculum delivery.

Tom Sandford BSc (Hons), Dip N, RGN, RMN
Tom Sandford is employed by the Royal College of Nursing (RCN) as the executive director of their services across England. His previous roles in the organisation include five years as a policy adviser and three years as London regional director. Before joining the RCN Tom was general manager of mental health services in the London boroughs of Camden and Islington.

Tom trained as a general and mental health nurse and held a variety of clinical posts in the fields of family therapy and acute and liaison psychiatry. He was Head of Professional Development in Bloomsbury Health Authority and was a member of the ministerial task force coordinating the development of the mental health national service framework. He has served on several public untoward incident inquiries and has taught mental health programmes at universities in Irsee and Frankfurt in Germany, and case management programmes at the University of Barcelona in Spain.

Contributors

Julie Attenborough RMN, BSc (Hons), MSc, PGCE (A) is a senior lecturer in the Educational Development Unit, School of Community and Health Sciences, City University London. Her background is in substance abuse, dual diagnosis and homelessness and mental health. She has an interest in the development and utilisation of e-learning tools in higher education and has been involved in the development and production of a CD-ROM for mental health workers in primary care and a DVD produced as an interprofessional training resource for medical and nursing students.

Linda Bailey RGN, PG Dip Community Health (health visiting), BA (Hons) Social Policy, MSc Public Health, FFPH is currently working as a public health consultant in east London. She is also a qualified nurse and health visitor and has a specialist interest in blood-borne viruses.

Hülya Bilgin PhD is assistant professor of psychiatric nursing in the Florence Nightingale School of Nursing at Istanbul University. Hulya trained as a nurse in Istanbul and completed first an M.Sc and then a PhD in psychiatric nursing. Since 1994, Hulya has been in the Department of Psychiatric Nursing at Istanbul University, Florence Nightingale School of Nursing as a lecturer, researcher and supervisor. Hulya's main interests concern aggression and violence in psychiatric care and community psychodrama and art therapy. She is an active member of the European Violence in Psychiatric Research Group and the Psychiatric Nurses Association in Turkey.

John Budd is a GP with the Edinburgh Homeless Practice. He has a clinical interest in substance misuse and a research interest in drug misuse and hepatitis C. John previously worked as a community doctor in rural South Africa, where he developed an interest in blood-borne viral illnesses and has since been involved in developing a GP exchange programme with the Western Cape Department of Health, South Africa.

Patrick Callaghan RN BSc, MSc, Ph.D., C.Psychol. CSci., FHEA is a mental health nurse and chartered health psychologist. He is professor of mental health nursing at the University of Nottingham, UK, and the Nottinghamshire NHS Healthcare Trust, where he heads a research programme designed to enable people to recover from mental distress, leading on service evaluation, testing the effect of psychosocial interventions on health and well-being and investigating links between mental health nursing and service user outcomes.

Melinda Campopiano is an attending physician in addiction medicine and family medicine in Pittsburgh, Pennsylvania. She is clinical faculty at the University of Pittsburgh Medical Center in both the psychiatry and family medicine departments where she teaches medical students and resident physicians. She is an alumnus of the University of Pittsburgh School of Medicine and the University of Iowa College of Liberal Arts. Dr Campopiano has been an invited speaker at national and international conferences where she has addressed topics from medication therapy in substance use disorders to harm reduction and biopsychosocial approaches to substance use disorder management. She is an activist for drug policy reform and community public health responses to substance-use-related problems such as overdose.

Dr Peter Carter OBE is the Chief Executive & General Secretary of the Royal College of Nursing (RCN), the world's largest professional union of nurses. The RCN has a membership of 400,000 nurses, midwives, health visitors, nursing students, cadets and health care assistants. Before assuming the post of RCN General Secretary in January 2007, Dr Carter spent almost twelve years as the Chief Executive of the Central and North West London Mental Health NHS Trust, one of the largest mental health trusts in the UK with an operating budget of over £200 million and an international reputation. He commenced his NHS career by training as a psychiatric nurse at Hill End Hospital, St Albans. He is also a general nurse, having trained at St Albans City Hospital and the Institute of Urology in London. In addition he has held a number of clinical and managerial posts in Hertfordshire, Bedfordshire and London. Dr Carter is a graduate, and a member, of the Chartered Institute of Personnel. He also has a Masters Degree in Business Administration and a PhD – both from the University of Birmingham. He was awarded the OBE for services to the NHS in the 2006 New Year's Honours. He has recently taken up a visiting professorship at the Florence Nightingale School of Nursing and Midwifery at King's College London.

Gary Croton RPN MHSc (AOD) is a psychiatric nurse and drug and alcohol specialist and has worked in mental health and drug treatment settings in Australia and the United Kingdom for over 30 years. Since 1998, Gary has been the sole worker for the Eastern Hume Dual Diagnosis Service, a rural Australian dual diagnosis capacity-building service. Eastern Hume Dual Diagnosis has used a range of innovative strategies to build the service system's capacity to contribute to better outcomes for persons with co-occurring mental health and substance use disorders. In 2004, Gary was awarded a Victorian Travelling Fellowship to investigate integrated treatment of co-occurring mental health and substance use disorders. Over a 6-week period, he conducted interviews with key informants in 22 site visits in the United Kingdom, United States and New Zealand. Gary serves on the current Victorian Ministerial Advisory Committee on Mental Health and is a member of the International Advisory Board for the new journal *Mental Health and Substance Use: Dual Diagnosis*. Gary has authored articles, submissions and conference papers around systemic, agency and clinician level responses to co-occurring disorders.

Sharon Dennis, RMN, BSc (Hons), CMS, RNT, Dip Family Therapy, Dip Performance Coaching (Business), PG Dip Advanced Practice (Nursing), is a regional director at the Royal College of Nursing (RCN). Prior to joining the RCN, Sharon has worked in London NHS mental health services for 20 years, culminating in a role as director of Nursing and Public Involvement and nurse adviser at the National Patient Safety Agency. Her publications include those on professional nursing issues and observation and she has a regular column in the *Nursing Standard* for whom she is the annual guest editor for their *Black History Month* special edition. She has contributed to Department of Health policy documents and National Institute for Clinical Excellence (NICE) guidance. She was an elected steering committee member of the

RCN's Mental Health Forum, a member of the RCN Mental Health Advisory Panel and Women's Mental Health Group and a nursing ambassador for the *Nursing Standard* magazine. Sharon job-shares at the RCN and has worked concurrently in professional leadership, commissioning, consultancy and project management roles.

Sue Excell, University London, UK, specialises in Dual Diagnosis and Older People. Susan supports students to evidence best practice through developing advanced portfolios of professional practice. She is a Service Manager for a Kent NHS Trust and provides specialised training to Health & Social Care professionals regarding Dual Diagnosis and policy development. She has recently supported Social Services to develop information leaflets for safer drinking in later life. Susan has also supported the Trust as a lead clinician in Practice Development.

Chris Glover is currently working as an alcohol liaison nurse at the Whittington Hospital. She has worked in the substance misuse field for over 20 years. Her career includes holding the positions of clinical services manager and lead nurse for substance misuse services, both at Camden and Islington Foundation NHS Trust. She has also held the position of lecturer/practitioner on the dual diagnosis programmes at Middlesex University.

Kevin Gournay is a chartered psychologist, chartered scientist and a registered nurse. Originally he trained in psychiatry, learning disabilities and general nursing and then, in the 1970s as one of the first nurse therapists in cognitive behaviour therapy. He worked part time to obtain a qualification as a psychologist, obtaining his PhD in agoraphobia. For the last 30 years, he has combined roles as a clinician treating people with post-traumatic stress and anxiety disorders, depression and psychosis; a researcher; a teacher and a policy advisor to various governments. He has published over 300 papers, chapters and books and made numerous contributions to television and radio. He has worked on a range of dual diagnosis research, education and policy projects over a 15-year period. He is the president and founding patron of No Panic, the United Kingdom's largest anxiety disorders charity. Among various honours he held, he is a Fellow of the Royal College of Psychiatrists, a Fellow of the Academy of Medical Science, a Fellow of the Royal College of Nursing and was elected Nurse of the Year by the American Psychiatric Nursing Association in 2004. He was appointed CBE in the Queen's New Year's Honours 1999. He retired from the Institute of Psychiatry, Kings College, London, in 2006 and in semi-retirement works as a clinician and an expert witness. He retains involvement in a dual diagnosis project at the National Drug and Alcohol Research Centre in Sydney, Australia.

Liz Hughes is reader in applied research in the Faculty of Health and Life Sciences at the University of Coventry. Liz is a mental health nurse by background and has worked in acute mental health and substance misuse services in London. She worked as a dual diagnosis worker, prior to obtaining a teaching and research post at the Institute of Psychiatry in 1999. This role involves leading the dual diagnosis programme as well as two major research trials of dual diagnosis training, and a London-wide dual diagnosis training dissemination project. Liz has completed a PhD in health services research during this time at King's College, London. Liz moved to the Centre for Clinical and Academic Workforce Innovation at the University of Lincoln in 2005, where she developed the area of dual diagnosis in relation to the criminal justice system and has delivered and evaluated training in London prisons. Liz has been commissioned by the National Institute for Mental Health in England (NIMHE) national programme for dual diagnosis to develop a number of products for national dissemination, including a CD-ROM of training materials and a capabilities framework for dual diagnosis.

Sonia Johnson studied social and political sciences and medicine at the Universities of Oxford and Cambridge, and also has an MSc in social psychology from the London School of Economics and a DM degree from the University of Oxford. She trained in psychiatry at the Bethlem Royal and Maudsley Hospitals, and was a lecturer in community psychiatry at the Institute of Psychiatry. Since 1997, she has worked at University College London (UCL) and in Camden and Islington Foundation Trust, and she is now a professor of social and community psychiatry at UCL. Dual diagnosis has been one of her major research interests for some years. She managed one of the first UK epidemiological investigations of dual diagnosis, and subsequently the COMO trial of training in management of dual diagnosis for care coordinators. She has supervised students working on ethnic differences and on motivations for use in dual diagnosis, and is currently involved in research on cannabis use in first episode psychosis.

David Jones is a lecturer in mental health and social care in the School of Nursing, Midwifery and Physiotherapy at the University of Nottingham. He is a mental health nurse whose clinical background is in both mental health and substance misuse.

Rob Keukens is a mental health consultant at the Global Initiative on Psychiatry and lecturer at HAN University, Nijmegen, the Netherlands.

Kathleen Leo PMHCNS-BC is currently a PhD candidate at Seton Hall University College of Nursing. She received her bachelor of science from

Rutgers University College of Nursing and her master of science from Rutgers Graduate School in advanced psychiatric and mental health nursing practice. She is a recipient of the Sigma Theta Tau Excellence in Scholarship Awards, the Marcia Granucci Memorial Scholarship and the RN Excellence in Nursing Award. She has been a three-time recipient of the New Jersey Department of Health, Division of Addiction Services Scholarship, receiving Certificates from the Rutgers Institute of Alcohol and Drug Studies. She has been appointed to several local and State of New Jersey boards, including governor-appointed board of trustee, Woodbridge Developmental Center and the State Medical Assistance Advisory Board. She attends the Philadelphia School of Psychoanalysis, Philadelphia, PA, and is in private practice in Matawan, NJ.

Simon McArdle is a senior lecturer in mental health at the University of Greenwich, London, UK. He has a clinical background working with patients with personality disorder in forensic mental health services and therapeutic communities. He is an ex-member of the executive committee of the Association of Therapeutic Communities and is currently reviews editor of the *International Journal of Therapeutic Communities*.

Jenny Oates is a lecturer in mental health at City University London. Her professional background is as a community mental health nurse and a psychiatric liaison nurse. Her academic interests include finding ways to narrow the gap between policy and practice, with particular reference to risk assessment and management, the care programme approach and supporting the physical health needs of people with mental illness.

She is currently working with other colleagues at City University on a study of violence and aggression in renal settings, and on a project looking at how in-patient staff can support the parenting needs of in-patient mental health service users.

Lisa Reynolds is a lecturer in mental health at City University London. She is a registered mental health nurse and has experience of working in forensic and acute mental health services. Her teaching and research interests include forensic mental health care, risk assessment and management within mental health services. In her role as a lecturer in mental health, Lisa works in partnership with mental health services users to develop and deliver learning activities, including the creation of reusable learning objects. Previous educational and research activities include the development of an online discussion forum with mental health service users and student nurses. Currently, Lisa is a doctoral research fellow undertaking an observational study of a medium secure unit. She is also a co-convenor of the British Sociological Association (BSA) risk group.

Jane Salvage, RGN, BA, MSc, Hon LLD, is an independent health care consultant and visiting professor at the Florence Nightingale School of Nursing and Midwifery, King's College, University of London, England. She has worked extensively on nursing development in eastern Europe and the former Soviet Union, as well as at home in the United Kingdom. From 2001 to 2006 she was a member of the board of the Global Initiative on Psychiatry (GIP), managed a major GIP project on mental health and HIV/AIDS and is a founder member of the GIP network for mental health nurses.

Lorna Saunder graduated from the University of Abertay, Dundee, in 1996 with a BSc (Hons) in Nursing, Mental Health. She left Scotland and returned to England to work in acute psychiatric services. Lorna then briefly worked in a mother and baby unit before eventually deciding that she wanted to pursue a career in helping people with substance use problems. She worked both in residential detoxification and community services. An opportunity then arose for Lorna to combine her clinical skills and a more academic role when she became lecture practitioner in dual diagnosis. Lorna has a PG diploma in academic practice and a PG diploma in drug and alcohol studies.

Theodora Sirota is associate professor of nursing at Seton Hall University College of Nursing, South Orange, NJ, a psychodynamic psychotherapist in private practice, and a group facilitator for the New Jersey State Nurses' Association Recovery and Maintenance Program (RAMP), working with nurses who have substance abuse problems. She received a diploma in nursing from The Mt Sinai Hospital School of Nursing, New York, NY, a BS degree in nursing, an MA in psychiatric mental health nursing of adults, and a PhD degree in nursing research, all from New York University, New York, NY. Theo is certified in psychoanalytic psychotherapy by the National Institute for the Psychotherapies, New York, NY, and holds certifications as clinical nurse leader from the American Association of Colleges of Nursing (AACN) and as a Psychiatric Mental Health Clinical Nurse Specialist-Board Certified from the American Nurses' Credentialing Center (ANCC).

Murat Soncul trained as a dental surgeon in Turkey, after which he completed a PhD in oral and maxillofacial surgery at University College London. He became interested in drug user oral health issues while working as a research fellow. His interests include health technology that improves access to services and assists diagnosis and treatment outcomes. Murat currently works with South London and Maudsley NHS Trust.

David Webb completed the world's first PhD on suicide as someone who has attempted suicide. In his thesis he argued that suicide is best understood as a crisis of the self rather than the prevailing view that it is the consequence of some pseudoscientific 'mental illness'. Prior to his PhD in 2006 (and the 'four years of madness' that motivated this research), David worked in the computer industry as a software developer and university lecturer. He has been a board member of the World Network of Users and Survivors of Psychiatry (WNUSP) and currently works part time as a research/policy officer with the Australia Federation of Disability Organisations. He regards human rights as the core issue in mental health and that justice will not be possible for users and survivors of psychiatry until the mental health industry moves to the social model of disability that is the basis of the UN Convention on the Rights of Persons with Disability. He has lived in New York, Delhi and London and now lives among the gum trees and kookaburras on the edge of Melbourne as he learns how to be a grandad without having ever been a dad.

Julie Winnington has worked in the addiction field for a number of years, both in the community and in in-patient settings. She currently works for the South London and Maudsley NHS Foundation Trust, managing an in-patient unit for drug and alcohol users in crisis. She has a special interest in women with dual diagnosis.

Foreword

The past decade has seen substantial clinical and research activity relating to the challenges presented by service users with a 'dual diagnosis'. We understand a lot more about the prevalence of substance misuse among the severely mentally ill and the interventions that might be effective in helping people with a dual diagnosis. This emphasis on effective clinical management is critical. As the chief executive of an inner London mental health NHS Trust between 1995 and 2007, I witnessed the rapidly rising incidence of service users with a dual diagnosis in our in-patient units. They have special needs and are often a highly disadvantaged population, impacted by the stigma of mental illness and that associated with drug-related problems. They frequently get a bad press in mental health services, where illicit drug use on in-patient areas has been the source of considerable concern. Drug-related deaths are too frequent and generate much sadness.

The investment that has been made into training and developing the confidence of staff working with people with a dual diagnosis has been welcome. Some good progress has been made around designing specific and appropriate services. However, there is still much more to do in terms of ensuring that this provision is able to respond in sustainable, creative and engaging ways to people with a dual diagnosis.

This book is a welcome step towards that journey. It attempts to understand the dynamics of substance misuse for service users and service providers. It brings together a good cross section of contributors with clinical, academic and policy backgrounds and many different perspectives are expressed. It captures the resourcefulness and energy of some of the great people that we have working in this field, and I hope that it will stimulate the next generation of clinicians and researchers who contribute to developing our knowledge base and skills still further.

Peter Carter OBE, PhD, MBA, MCIPD, RGN, RMN

Part 1

Contemporary Context

Chapter 1

Definition, Recognition and Assessment

Olive McKeown

Introduction

Dual diagnosis is arguably one of the most significant problems facing health services. A significant percentage of all patients in general hospitals are thought to be there because of complications related to alcohol consumption, and many people who misuse alcohol and other substances are thought to have at least one mental illness. The relevant literature supports the hypothesis that mental illness and substance misuse occur together more frequently than chance would predict (Lehman *et al.* 2000).

Substance misuse and mental health problems individually constitute a challenging area of work for health care professionals. In combination, these problems place considerable demands on health services and on individual practitioners, often stretching resources and the skills of professionals to their limits. There has been a growing awareness in the United States for some time that there is an increasing pattern of the coexistence or co-occurrence of mental health and substance misuse problems (Regier *et al.* 1990). More recently, in the United Kingdom, awareness about the seriousness of dual diagnosis has been reflected in several Department of Health papers/guidelines. At about the same time, research and publications as well as university-based theory and skills programmes have been established in some parts of the United Kingdom.

The Task Force review was produced in May 1996 by the Department of Health (1996) as part of the government's drug strategy. This was an in-depth review of the effectiveness of treatment for drug misusers in this country. In the report there is recognition of the problem of dual diagnosis, and one of its recommendations is as follows:

> *Purchasers and providers should ensure that people working in both drugs and mental illness services are aware of the need to identify and respond to problems of combined psychiatric illness and drug misuse.*

3

A few years later, The National Service Framework (NSF) for Mental Health (Department of Health 1999), while emphasising the importance of tackling management of dual diagnosis, failed to include standards and service models to address the challenges posed by patients with dual diagnosis, including those with severe mental illness. It was in the context of this gap in policy that the *Dual Diagnosis Good Practice Guide* (Department of Health 2002) was launched. Notably, the NSF also failed to provide standards and to suggest service models for people with substance use disorders, an omission that was addressed by the complementary guidance on models of care produced by the National Treatment Agency (2002) for substance misuse. Since then, recognition and awareness of dual diagnosis in the United Kingdom appears to have grown substantially although dual diagnosis practice guidelines published in 2002 and 2006 have been regarded as being 'toothless tigers' because of their respective lack of directives and financial incentives or drivers for service providers. The existing gaps within practice and service delivery are compounded and perhaps caused to some extent by the dearth of curriculum coverage within basic medical and nursing training.

Definition and terminology

Defining dual diagnosis is a challenge because of its complex and multifaceted nature. A simple definition would be that it is a combination of a mental illness and substance misuse problem co-occurring in one person. Personality disorder may also coexist with mental illness or substance misuse. The term originated from the United States in the 1980s and was adopted in the United Kingdom more recently. The nature of the relationship between the two conditions is complex and is sometimes controversial.

Some authors such as McKeown and Derricott (1996) have argued against the use of the term 'dual diagnosis', noting the necessity that health care workers need to pay attention to the language they use in every day practice. They express concern that with the use of the term dual diagnosis and the adoption of a wholly medical philosophy, patients may become disadvantaged, with the understanding of and the potential solutions to problems getting limited. Rostad and Checinski (1996) also debate the usefulness of the term dual diagnosis, suggesting that it is 'labelling of the worst kind'. They argue so despite bearing in mind that the label in itself serves a very useful purpose in drawing attention to a very real problem, which is not generally well addressed in the United Kingdom.

Abou-Saleh (2004) suggests that 'comorbidity' might be a better term, although he does not explain his reasons for this view. The term comorbidity is being widely used internationally in the last few years and is gradually gaining popularity in the United Kingdom. In essence, the shift to using this term simply represents a direct translation from English to a Latin medically orientated term, with very little advantage apart from the possible medical-isation or perhaps mystification of the term, which arguably is of dubious advantage. It may be that professionals interested in improving the plight of patients with dual diagnosis are replacing one label that is perceived by some as having become unhelpful or counter-productive with one associated more closely with an illness model, perhaps in an attempt to shift blame or responsibility away from individual patients and implicitly suggesting that patients are treatable, thereby endeavouring to promote more optimism about potential treatment outcomes.

General considerations in the recognition and assessment of dual diagnosis

Assessment and diagnosis of patients should be driven by practitioners' intention to make practical and helpful judgements about patients' diagno-sis and subsequently to liaise and communicate with each other to work towards effective collaborative management and treatment. Patients may need a variety of approaches to assessment and diagnosis at different stages of presentation and treatment. Initially, it is important to recognise that both problems exist concomitantly and practitioners should avoid coming to premature conclusions about which diagnosis is primary and which is sec-ondary. Longer term management and treatment may necessitate systematic re-evaluation about why a patient has developed both disorders.

A common issue in diagnosing and classifying dual diagnosis patients is that generally there remains a lack of knowledge and awareness about the nature of patients' problems and what strategies and approaches are most helpful. This lack of clarity makes it difficult for practitioners to identify what exactly needs to be prioritised for assessment and subsequent treat-ment. Understandably, lack of knowledge and awareness on the part of practitioners has major implications for the recognition of dual diagnosis in the first instance. These circumstances further support the need for improv-ing undergraduate training for health professionals about substance misuse and dual diagnosis.

How significant is the problem of dual diagnosis?

The National Institute of Mental Health's Epidemiologic Catchment Area (ECA) study (Regier *et al.* 1990) provided important information on lifetime prevalence of substance misuse and mental health problems within the population generally. In the United Kingdom, it is thought that the number of people with a potential dual diagnosis is high and may be increasing. Com-munity Mental Health Trusts typically report that 8–15% of their patients have dual diagnosis problems, but rates appear higher in inner cities. One UK survey showed that 36% of patients seen by an inner London psychiatric service were dependent on alcohol and/or drugs (Menezes *et al.* 1996). Farrell *et al.* (2001), in a UK national household survey, reported prevalence rates of psychiatric disorder of 22% in nicotine dependence, 30% in alcohol dependence and 45% in drug dependence, compared with 12% prevalence in the non-dependent population. The National Confidential Inquiry into Suicide and Homicide has reported substance misuse as a factor in more than 50% of homicides and suicides by people with serious mental illness (Department of Health 2001). In addition, it is noteworthy that this group has high rates of criminality and blood-borne infections, including HIV infection and hepatitis B and C.

Work carried out in New Hampshire has shown that patients with dual diagnosis make considerably more demands on health and social services (Drake *et al.* 1993), which is corroborated by the London survey (Menezes *et al.* 1996), indicating that patients in this group spent almost twice as long in hospital as people without a substance misuse problem. The experience of work in this area in the United States indicates that effective management of dual diagnosis entails integrating approaches to both mental illness and substance misuse. In most countries, the integration of services is proving to be difficult in practice as mental health and substance misuse services frequently tend to operate very differently, and usually quite separately, with their own unique cultures.

Recognition and assessment

The severity of mental illness in people who seek treatment for substance misuse is a good predictor of substance misuse outcomes, as more severe symptoms predict poorer outcomes. Outcomes for mental health patients with a substance misuse disorder are typically poorer than outcomes for mental health patients without a substance problem. This point in itself underlines the importance or even the necessity of health services and clinicians working towards improved approaches and services for dual diagnosis patients.

During the initial period of contact, general observation, withdrawal management, and the treatment of acute mental health symptoms are important to help regain a degree of stability. From the outset, the possibility that the patient has both substance-related and mental health problems should be considered, given the commonality of both. It is important to ascertain whether mental health symptoms begin to improve as detoxification or withdrawal progresses. In situations where mental health symptoms diminish completely once patients have completed the detoxification process and where the patient has no prior history of mental illness, dual diagnosis is very unlikely. If, on the other hand, the mental symptoms persist after detoxification is complete or if there is a clear history of previous mental illness, dual diagnosis should be carefully considered as a possibility.

During the initial phase of observation and assessment, there is often a tendency for practitioners to miss or fail to recognise the possibility of both problems or mistake the symptoms of one of the disorders for the other. When practitioners lack knowledge and skill in either mental health- or substance-related presentations, patients will inevitably receive less than optimal management and care. Early recognition would lead to improvement in helping patients understand the nature of their problems and enhance their willingness to consider useful treatment options. Patients' response to treatment options and subsequent engagement is heavily influenced by the quality of information provided, and on whether or not they have a degree of choice about management and interventions. Providing patients with choice and involving them in decision making from the outset whenever possible increases a sense of empowerment and respect and, in the longer term, is likely to enhance motivation.

Another issue related to initial assessment is the tendency to assume the primacy of either the mental health or the substance-related problem. There is a general agreement within the literature that this phase of treatment should include the integration of assessment and treatment for both disorders. The integrated approach seems to lead to a more effective treatment experience for patients with dual diagnosis who are so often passed between services, with services providers in disagreement about which problem is primary, often refusing to treat the patient until they demonstrate 'stability'. There is some debate about whether patients can be treated satisfactorily while being engaged simultaneously with more than one treatment programme or whether specialist dual diagnosis treatment programmes are necessary. The priority is to identify and treat all presenting symptoms as cohesively as possible as early as possible (McKeown 2004).

Main stream mental health services are arguably best placed to offer an integrated approach, but to be effective mental health staff require considerable support, education and ongoing training. A crucial element of support for staff must come from staff in management and leadership roles and therefore managers of services also need to have suitable training, particularly related to developing more positive attitudes towards dual diagnosis patients (McKeown 2004). Lack of optimism among senior staff is not conducive to encouraging those in key clinical roles to become interested and confident in working on dual diagnosis.

For many reasons, it can be difficult for practitioners to be consistently confident or clear about which patients have a dual diagnosis. The challenge is to establish when the use of psychoactive substances constitutes 'misuse' among mental health patients and when the symptoms of mental illness among substance misusers should be considered to constitute a mental illness? It is difficult to establish where the line should be drawn or even whether drawing such a line is helpful, ethical or valid.

Some examples of clinical presentation that could be difficult to categorise as being clearly dual diagnostic are given below:

- A patient who uses amphetamines, from time to time, develops psychotic symptoms and appears depressed during periods when he or she is not using stimulants
- A patient who is dependent on alcohol and develops key symptoms of schizophrenia while withdrawing from alcohol
- A patient who suffers from an episode of major depression and drinks alcohol when he or she is depressed
- A patient who suffers from a bipolar illness and drinks when he or she has a manic episode

Considering the tendency for practitioners to overlook or fail to recognise dual diagnosis, it is important for service managers, educators of health care professionals and practice protocols to encourage individual professionals to be constantly vigilant and aware that dual diagnosis, especially within mental health settings, is the norm and not the exception. Practitioners need to be supported and encouraged to conduct an in-depth assessment of both mental health and substance disorders because all patients resist making a decision about which problem or disorder is primary.

Hypotheses

1. *Mental illness is primary and substance misuse is secondary*

The patient suffers from a primary mental illness, and the symptoms and consequences of the illness or its treatment (e.g. side effects of medication) lead to addiction or substance dependence as a means of coping with mental illness. This view subscribes to the concept of self-medication and that secondary substance misuse is at least in part attributable to issues such as cognitive impairment and/or social passivity.

When appraising the literature related to risk factors for developing an addiction or drug dependence, it becomes clear that most of the risk factors identified are also present for a person with mental illness. Commonly cited risk factors for addiction or dependence include the following:

- Negative mood states
- Impaired cognition
- Poor social skills
- Poor sense of self-control and self-efficacy

- Poor role performance
- Poor self-esteem
- Lack of social support
- Limited coping skills

Having considered the above issues, it is not surprising that people who have a mental illness also have a high rate of substance misuse. The risk of actually developing an addiction or dependence problem per se may be increased as a result of the many psychosocial complications of having a mental illness. Problems and experiences such as low self-esteem, social and emotional isolation, unemployment and social exclusion could potentially entice an individual to seek refuge or comfort by using substances or perhaps to belong to a drug using sub-culture. This view does not necessarily embrace the notion that there is a clear association between a particular mental illness and the misuse of a specific substance.

Some mental illnesses may lead to patients using particular substances to alleviate the negative effects of their illness. There may be, for example, an association between stimulant use and some psychotic disorders. The use of alcohol and other depressant substances may be linked with mood disorders. The existing literature fails to report consistent and reliable associations between particular mental illnesses and specific substances and so the evidence, although interesting, so far remains speculative overall.

Cesarec and Nyman (1985) found differing responses to stimulants among subgroups of people with schizophrenia; patients with predominantly negative symptoms tended to improve when prescribed a combination of neuroleptic and stimulant medications, but patients with acute psychotic symptoms became worse with the same medication regime. Understanding the differences in substance use patterns among specific groups of dual diagnosis patients could, in the future, lead to the identification of physiologically or genetically heterogeneous subtypes of patients. DiSalver (1987) hypothesised that substances used typically by patients with affective disorders could provide clues to the pathologies of this type of disorder. He speculated that there may be an association between the use of anticholinergic substances and the monoamine model of affective disorders.

2.　*Primary substance misuse with psychiatric consequences*

This hypothesis suggests that the patient suffers primarily from a substance misuse problem and that the mental illness is a manifestation of the effects of the substances misused. For example, depression in the case of cocaine users and other stimulants users; or cognitive impairment and thought disorders related to alcohol misuse; or psychosis triggered by amphetamine-based substances or LSD. Also included in this hypothesis are acute mental illnesses linked with withdrawal and intoxication. These clinical presentations can usually improve when the patient completes a withdrawal/detoxification process.

It is not clear whether primary substance misuse can lead to enduring mental illness when substance use is not maintained. There is some evidence to support this hypothesis, such as chronic psychotic syndromes that arise as a result of long-term stimulants use.

There remains a debate about whether enduring mental illness follows primary substance misuse or whether it is the result of a pre-existing vulnerability to mental illness triggered by substance misuse or perhaps the long-term changes in the physiology of the brain caused by substance misuse. Patients whose presentations fit this hypothesis could benefit from rehabilitation in a substance treatment setting.

3.   A dual primary diagnosis

This hypothesis proposes that the patient suffers from two unrelated disorders that may interact to exacerbate each other. The seeming increase in the coexistence of mental illness and substance misuse tends to contradict this hypothesis. On the other hand, some subgroups of patients could arguably fit this hypothesis. Some studies have not found an excess incidence of alcoholic patients with schizophrenia, although this trend is not consistent in the wider literature.

The key concept within this model is that coexistence of primary mental illness and substance misuse problems may in themselves change the way either problem actually presents clinically, thus making diagnosis and treatment considerably more challenging. The main implication of this hypothesis is that dually diagnosed patients who fit this model need treatment and ongoing care for both mental illness and substance use problems. Parallel treatment or, more ideally, integrated treatment for both sets of problems would be necessary.

4.   A common aetiology

This hypothesis posits that common underlying factors may predispose a patient both to mental illness and to substance use disorders. The most common example is the idea that alcohol dependency and affective disorders are common within some families, but there is a debate about whether this association points to a common underlying genetic cause or other issues, such as assortative mating.

Whether a genetic link exists or not, some dual diagnoses may have a common biologic aetiology. Some particular defects in dopamine function could predispose individuals to schizophrenic type illnesses and to the possibility of misusing dopamine agonists such as amphetamine. In a similar way, some defects in cholinergic activity could predispose individuals to mood disorders and drug misuse, impacting on cholinergic pathways.

There may of course also exist some common biopsychosocial factors that predispose susceptible individuals to both mental illness and substance misuse. One such example would be a person who becomes homeless and subsequently develops depression and a substance-related problem. The treatment implication associated with this hypothesis is that if such common underlying aetiologic factors exist, then treatment should be tailored to address these. A possible approach to intervention in this case will be to address and treat the mental illness and substance use, ideally in an integrated manner.

There are several identifiable recurrent themes in the dual diagnosis literature, for example, lack of awareness of the prevalence of dual diagnosis; lack of knowledge or skill in detection, assessment and management; negative attitudes towards substance users and mental health problems; inconsistency about definition and terminology; a dearth of suitable research instruments; blindness of clinicians in 'seeing' the problem; a need for closer liaison and collaboration between professionals; the value of an integrated model of care; frequent chronicity in the course of dual diagnosis and the attendant financial and social costs to the family, society and health services and an absence of recent research on dual diagnosis in acute general psychiatric in-patient settings in the United Kingdom.

Conclusion

An important message emerging from the existing literature and all but one of the clinical hypotheses discussed earlier is that dual diagnosis is not simply a statistical phenomenon of co-occurrence but is an interactive phenomenon that is putting mentally ill people at high risk for substance misuse and substance misusers at high risk for the development of a mental illness. The concept of dual diagnosis arises from the theoretical segregation of mental disorders and substance misuse within commonly used classification systems such as DSM IV and ICD-10. The existing conceptual duality makes little sense clinically. Many dual diagnosis patients suffer from multiple problems/disorders, so in reality dual diagnosis could be construed as a misleading and over-simplistic concept.

Although many existing service structures and facilities are less than ideal for the optimisation of care delivery for dual diagnosis patients, if individual practitioners are interested and adequately determined to improve their individual practice then undoubtedly some patients will benefit. Some recent improvements and initiatives to dual diagnosis services in the United Kingdom serve as examples and inspiration for others to follow, but further radical changes in funding, training and support mechanisms are necessary to transform the current status of dual diagnosis care and to ensure that these patients have fair access to appropriate treatment.

References

Abou-Saleh MT (2004) Dual diagnosis: management within a psychosocial context. *Advances in Psychiatric Treatment* 10: 352–360.

Cesarec Z, Nyman AK (1985) Differential response to amphetamine in schizophrenia. *Acta Psychiatrica Scandinavica* 71: 523–538.

Department of Health (1996) *The Task Force to Review Service for Drug Misusers.* Report of an Independent Review of Drug Treatment Services in England. London: Department of Health.

Department of Health (1999) *National Service Framework for Mental Health: Modern Standards and Service Models.* London: Department of Health.

Department of Health (2001) *Safety First: Five-year Report of the National Confidential Inquiry into Suicide and Homicide by People with Mental Illness.* London: Department of Health.

Department of Health (2002) *Dual Diagnosis Good Practice Guide.* London: Department of Health.

DiSalver SC (1987) The psychophysiologies of substance abuse and affective disorders: An integrative model? *Journal of Clinical Psychiatry* 43: 25–228.

Drake R, Bartels S, Teague G, Noordsy D, Clark R (1993) Treatment of substance abuse in severely mentally ill patients. *Journal of Nervous and Mental Disorders* 181: 606–611.

Farrell M, Howes S, Bebbington P, Brugha T, Jenkins R (2001) Nicotine, alcohol and drug dependence and psychiatric comorbidity. *British Journal of Psychiatry* 179: 432–437.

Lehman AF, Myers CP, Corty E (2000) Assessment and classification of patients with psychiatric and substance abuse syndromes. *Psychiatric Services* 51 (9): 1119–1125.

McKeown O (2004) Dual diagnosis: a challenge for acute mental health nursing. Unpublished PhD thesis, Canterbury Christ Church University.

McKeown M, Derricott J (1996) Muddy waters. *Nursing Times* 92 (28): 30–31.

Menezes PR, Johnson S, Thornicroft G, *et al.* (1996) Drug and alcohol problems among people with severe mental illness in South London. *British Journal of Psychiatry* 168: 612–619.

National Treatment Agency (2002) *Models of Care for Treatment of Adult Drug Misusers.* London: Department of Health. http://www.nta.nhs.uk/publications/documents/nta_modelsofcare1_2002_moc1.pdf.

Regier D, Farmer N, Rae D (1990) Co-morbidity of mental disorders with alcohol and other drugs of abuse: results from the Epidemiological Catchment Area Study (ECAS). *Journal of the American Medical Association* 264: 2511–2518.

Rostad P, Checinski K (1996) *Dual Diagnosis: Facing the Challenge. The Care of People with a Dual Diagnosis of Mental Illness and Substance Misuse.* Surrey: Wynne Howard Publishing.

Chapter 2

Explanatory Models for Dual Diagnosis

Peter Phillips and Sonia Johnson

Introduction

Our aim in this chapter is to define a set of questions that are useful in attempting to understand the aetiology and development of co-morbid substance misuse or dependence and severe mental illness ('dual diagnosis') and to review the literature relevant to each of these. We will summarise the current evidence on each of these questions and consider what further research may need to be undertaken. Dual diagnosis has been defined in a variety of ways: this chapter will follow many papers in defining dual diagnosis relatively narrowly as the comorbidity of functional psychotic illness (including schizophrenia, schizoaffective disorder and manic depressive illness) and harmful substance use or dependence. Much of the research evidence concerns schizophrenia only so that this is the main emphasis of this chapter, but evidence regarding other psychotic illnesses has been included where available. One of the most relevant questions in regard to the development of dual diagnosis relates to whether substance use independently leads to functional psychotic illness.

The past 20 years have seen substantial clinical and research activity relating to the problems presented by service users with a 'dual diagnosis'. The resulting literature focuses on the prevalence of substance misuse among the severely mentally ill, its social and clinical correlates and the interventions that might be effective in people with a dual diagnosis. This emphasis on prevalence and clinical management seems to be predicated on an acceptance that the two problems do coexist and therefore need to be addressed in combination, without it being necessary to investigate how comorbidity has developed or which problem has arisen first. Once both problems are present, treatment will often need to address both so that this approach is pragmatic, but it leaves substantial questions unanswered in trying to understand the aetiology and context of development of dual diagnosis. Formulation of an explanatory model or models for the development of this comorbidity is desirable as a potentially fruitful source of preventive and therapeutic strategies.

Epidemiological, social, psychological and neurobiological levels of explanation may each be useful in seeking to understand dual diagnosis. The set of questions examined subsequently encompasses each of these levels and has been formulated so as to address each of the main forms of explanation of dual diagnosis so far proposed. The various possible explanations are not mutually exclusive, and it is probable that more than one aetiological factor is important.

Is substance misuse more prevalent among people with psychotic illnesses than in the general population?

This epidemiological question is an important starting point, as specific explanations for dual diagnosis would only be necessary if people with schizophrenia and other psychotic illnesses are more likely than the general population to misuse substances. If rates of substance use among people with psychotic illness were similar to those in the general population, it might be assumed that the important aetiological factors were probably similar to those in the population as a whole. One of the largest epidemiological investigations has been the Epidemiological Catchment Area (ECA) survey in the United States (Regier *et al.* 1990). In this study, 47% of subjects with schizophrenia (or schizophreniform disorder) showed evidence of current or past substance misuse, compared with general population rates of 13.5% for alcohol misuse and 6.1% for drug misuse. The odds ratio obtained when rates of substance misuse among individuals with schizophrenia were compared with the US population was 4.6, strongly suggesting a raised rate in people with these illnesses. A limitation of the ECA study, however, is that these comparisons do not take into account potentially confounding socio-demographic factors.

The authors of two major reviews regarding the epidemiology of dual diagnosis conclude that alcohol abuse is no more frequent in people with schizophrenia than in the general population but that stimulant abuse is more prevalent (Schneier & Siris 1987; Mueser *et al.* 1995). Schneier and Siris (1987) reviewed 18 US and UK studies undertaken between 1960 and 1986, and found broad agreement that people with schizophrenia were more likely than control subjects to use amphetamines, cocaine, cannabis and hallucinogens, but less likely to use alcohol, opiates and sedative hypnotics. A significant limitation of this review, however, is that, with one exception, the control groups in the studies reviewed consisted of in-patients and outpatients in treatment for other psychiatric disorders. The conclusion from a review by Mueser *et al.* (1995) is that substance misuse is not more prevalent in people with severe mental illnesses than in the general population, except for significantly raised rates of amphetamine and hallucinogen misuse. The evidence reviewed in this paper suggests that rates of cannabis, sedative, alcohol and narcotic abuse were lower than those of the general population as compared with the US national household survey on drug abuse. However, this survey used self-report of substance use, as opposed to the structured measures of DSM III-R substance abuse disorder or reports by key informants that are often used in studies of clinical populations.

An early UK study was carried out by Bernadt and Murray (1986), who compared adult patients admitted to an inner London hospital with a general population survey carried out in the same area. Psychiatric in-patients did not appear to have higher total alcohol consumption than the local population, and those with schizophrenia appeared to be drinking significantly less than either subjects with other psychiatric diagnoses and than the local general population. In the UK National Psychiatric Morbidity Survey (Farrell *et al.* 1998), drug and alcohol use was studied in three samples: a general population sample, an 'institutional' sample and a group of homeless individuals. Not enough individuals with schizophrenia were picked up in the household sample to make valid comparisons with the general population regarding patterns of substance use, but in the 'institutional' sample, people with schizophrenia were more likely than the general population to be abstinent from alcohol and less likely to be heavy drinkers, as defined in the study (household population heavy drinkers 5%, residents with schizophrenia 2%). With regard to drug use, the household population rate for any drug use in the past year was 5%, as opposed to the residents with schizophrenia who had a rate of 7%. However, people with schizophrenia living in sheltered settings may be markedly different from those living in the community, as substance misuse may be a bar to entry to sheltered accommodation and closely monitored and proscribed within such settings. Elsewhere in Europe, the limited epidemiological work so far available suggests that prevalence and patterns of substance misuse vary substantially from country to country, with studies carried out in countries including Germany (Soyka *et al.* 1993), France (Verdoux *et al.* 1996) and Switzerland (Modestin *et al.* 1997), suggesting that prevalence is not uniformly as high as in the United States and that opiate use is more frequent than stimulant use in some European subjects with schizophrenia. This evidence of large national variations is important in that it suggests that the mechanisms by which substance misuse develops among those with psychotic illness probably need to be understood in the context of local patterns of substance misuse and wider social and cultural factors influencing these.

Thus there is as yet no clear answer to the question of whether and how substance use patterns among those with schizophrenia really differ from those in the general population, with lack of comparable general population data being the main obstacle to drawing clear conclusions. It is also likely that patterns vary considerably between countries, but at least in the United States, it does appear probable that people with schizophrenia and other functional psychoses may have a particular propensity for stimulant use.

Which problem generally develops first in dual diagnosis?

An understanding of the temporal relationship between onset of substance misuse and of schizophrenia would be useful to understanding aetiology. If substance misuse were found generally to be present before the psychosis, this would make explanations in terms of self-medication less plausible and those invoking the concept of drug-induced psychosis more plausible. If schizophrenia tends to occur first, this would be compatible with explanations involving self-medication or the social circumstances of the mentally ill as causes of substance misuse.

Mueser *et al.* (1998) draw attention to the difficulties in establishing temporal sequence. The insidious characteristic onset of both substance misuse and schizophrenia makes the beginning of each difficult to pinpoint, and the retrospective methods of data collection used in most studies compound this difficulty. Silver and Abboud (1994) used first admission as the marker of onset of mental illness and retrospective self-report as a marker of onset of drug use. They reported that 60% of subjects with schizophrenia who used drugs had begun doing so before their first admission, although it remains unclear how long subjects had experienced psychotic symptoms before this admission. The conclusion that drug use more often develops before the onset of schizophrenia or during the prodromal phase of the illness is supported by other studies (Turner & Tsuang 1990; Kovasznay *et al.* 1993). Hambrecht and Hafner (1996) report a retrospective assessment of 232 people with schizophrenia in Germany, among whom a third already appeared to have had a drug problem for at least a year when schizophrenic illness began, while for a further third the two problems began within a year of each other, and for the final third the drug problem clearly occurred after the prodromal symptoms of schizophrenia. They also report that drug use tends to start slightly later in people with schizophrenia than in the general population, suggesting that drug use is unlikely to be the main direct cause of psychosis. From a study of first onset psychosis patients that compared subjects with a psychotic illness and no lifetime substance diagnosis, Rabinowitz *et al.* (1998) report subjects in remission from substance abuse or reporting mild drug use (with a co-morbid psychotic illness) and subjects with a co-morbid psychotic illness who reported moderate or severe substance abuse. The study found that in almost all those with a history of moderate to severe substance abuse, this predated the onset of psychotic illness. It was also related to earlier onset of psychosis in females and was predictive of antisocial behaviour in both male and females. Addington and Addington (1998) report findings similar to those of Rabinowitz *et al.* (1998) with regard to age of onset of symptoms of psychotic illness: subjects with substance misuse and psychosis had been significantly younger at the age of onset than those with psychosis only and were also younger at the time of first psychiatric admission. Cantwell *et al.* (1999) investigated a group of 168 subjects with first episode of schizophrenia in the United Kingdom to establish prevalence and pattern of substance use and misuse and alcohol misuse. Thirty seven percentage of the sample met the criteria for drug use or misuse or alcohol misuse at their first presentation to services (although 27% had experienced psychotic symptoms for more than 1 month before this point). This figure is similar to that reported for a mixed community sample of individuals with psychotic illness in the United Kingdom by Menezes *et al.* (1996), suggesting that substance misuse may often evolve either at a very early stage in schizophrenia, or possibly, before the illness. In summary, there is some evidence that substantial numbers of people with schizophrenia may already be using drugs by the time of their first contact with specialist services, so that explaining substance use wholly in terms of severely ill subjects resorting to substance misuse as a form of self-medication may not be plausible. However, a particular barrier to drawing clear conclusions is the often very insidious nature of illness onset, which makes temporal order very hard to establish. Prospective studies of individuals identified as being at high risk of developing psychotic illnesses or follow-up of cohorts of people who misuse substances might go some way towards clarifying the relationship between the onsets of psychosis and substance misuse.

Does dual diagnosis have a neurobiological basis?

There is some consensus that genetic factors have a role in both schizophrenia and alcohol misuse disorders, and increased rates of family history of alcohol disorders have been found among individuals with dual diagnosis compared with those with schizophrenia only (Noordsy *et al.* 1994). Thus, a possibility to be considered is whether this genetic vulnerability is to any degree a shared one between the two disorders. However, conflicting findings have been reported and it has not been clearly established that there is an increased vulnerability to psychotic illness among the relatives of individuals with drug and alcohol disorders or vice versa (Bidaut-Russell *et al.* 1994). The relationship of dual diagnosis to genetic factors has been fully discussed by Mueser *et al.* (1998), who conclude that at present the available evidence does not support the idea of a common genetic basis for substance misuse and functional psychotic illness. In considering the possibility of a biological explanation for the co-occurrence of functional psychotic illness and substance misuse, it is also worth noting that the dopaminergic neurotransmitter system features prominently in explanations for each (Amara & Sonders 1998; Fadda & Rossetti 1998; Harrison 1999). However, convincing aetiological models based on this do not, as yet, seem to have been put forward.

Is dual diagnosis mediated by personality disorder?

A further hypothesis concerning the aetiology of comorbidity between psychotic illness and substance misuse concerns the idea that individuals may have a common vulnerability to the two disorders, which is mediated by a third factor. Thus far, research in this area has concentrated on antisocial personality disorder. Personality disorders and substance misuse have long been observed to be associated (Nace *et al.* 1990; Dackis & Gold 1992; Campbell *et al.* 1993) and this is supported by evidence from the ECA survey (Regier *et al.* 1990), which reports a rate of severe substance misuse of more than 80% among people with antisocial personality disorder. An earlier onset of substance misuse in persons with antisocial personality disorder than in other substance misusers has also been reported (Johnston *et al.* 1978). A number of links have been reported between psychotic illness and antisocial personality disorder and are consistent with the idea that antisocial personality disorder may be a risk factor for both psychotic illness and substance misuse and thus explain high rates of comorbidity. In particular, features of conduct disorder (the childhood precursor of antisocial personality disorder) have been linked with the development of schizophrenia, bipolar disorder and substance misuse in adulthood (Neumann *et al.* 1995) and a shared genetic vulnerability to antisocial personality disorder, and schizophrenia remains a possibility (Mueser *et al.* 1998). Further research has also demonstrated that people with functional psychotic illness and antisocial personality disorder are more likely to have substance misuse problems than similar people with a functional psychotic illness alone (Caton 1995). Despite this, evidence for the role of antisocial personality disorder as a risk factor (for substance misuse in patients with a dual diagnosis) remains unclear; in particular, diagnostic uncertainties may relate to the difficulty in separating out antisocial personality disordered behaviour that is consequent to substance misuse itself, as opposed to it having a role as a risk factor for substance misuse in this population. Further to this, accurate assessment of the premorbid personality of individuals with schizophrenia or other functional psychotic illnesses remains particularly difficult because of the often early appearance of prodromal features of psychosis, thereby complicating the diagnosis of antisocial personality disorder in persons with functional psychotic illness. A full discussion of recent research relating to common factor models in the development of dual diagnosis has been undertaken by Mueser *et al.* (1998).

Do people with schizophrenia use substances as a form of self-medication?

The self-medication hypothesis suggests that people with functional psychotic illnesses initiate and continue drug and alcohol use as a direct consequence of their illness experience (Khantzian 1985; Phillips 1998). Several North American researchers have investigated self-reported motivations for and effects of alcohol and drug use among the severely mentally ill. Previously, Dixon *et al.* (1990) investigated 83 in-patients with diagnoses of schizophrenia, and schizoaffective and schizophreniform disorders admitted to a New York hospital over a 6-month period. The drugs most frequently used were cannabis, cocaine and alcohol. The most frequent self-reported reasons for use were to increase happiness and decrease depression and anxiety. Subjects also described using drugs to medicate positive symptoms such as hallucinations and suspiciousness, to counteract extrapyramidal side effects of medication and to alleviate negative symptoms such as apathy and lack of motivation. Addington and Duchak (1997) report from a study of out-patients with schizophrenic illness that substances were more often used to relieve dysphoria and anxiety and to alleviate tension and increase pleasure than for any direct effects on positive symptoms. Noordsy *et al.* (1991) investigated subjective experiences of alcohol use among a community sample of 75 people with schizophrenic illnesses in New Hampshire. They found that over two-thirds of the subjects identified their main motivation for alcohol use as relief of social anxiety and tension. Pristach and Smith (1996) reported the primary motivation for drinking among people with schizophrenia as relief of depressive symptoms. In both studies more than 50% of the subjects also reported positive effects of alcohol in alleviating apathy and anhedonia and improving sleep. Reports regarding effects on positive symptoms in these studies were mixed, with similar numbers reporting exacerbating and relieving effects. Baigent *et al.* (1995) report similar findings from a New Zealand study of in-patients with schizophrenia and substance misuse, the major self-reported motivations for substance use among people with schizophrenia being for its activating effects and as a reliever of dysphoria and anxiety in those with schizophrenia.

Taken together, evidence that relief of negative symptoms such as anhedonia and apathy is often a self-reported motivation for substance use and the data suggesting that people with schizophrenia may be particularly likely to use stimulants (discussed earlier) have formed the basis for a hypothesis that people with schizophrenia tend to use stimulants as a specific form of self-medication for negative symptoms. In relation to this possibility, Serper *et al.* (1996) report from a longitudinal study that compared cocaine-using subjects with schizophrenic illness with non-cocaine-using subjects with schizophrenia at presentation to the emergency psychiatric service and then after 3 weeks in hospital. Serper *et al.* (1996) found that the cocaine-using subjects reported significantly fewer negative symptoms than the non-cocaine-using subjects at first assessment and that at retest the negative symptoms were similar in both groups. This finding could be explained in terms of the effects of cocaine in relieving negative symptoms at the time of first assessment. However, it contrasts with the report by Dixon *et al.* (1990) of similar clinical pictures at the time of admission among schizophrenic subjects with and without drug abuse, followed by greater symptomatic improvement (of both positive and negative symptoms) during admission among the drug-using subjects. The beneficial effects of abstinence from drugs are put forward as a possible explanation for this finding.

Medication side effects have also been proposed as a possible target for self-medication. Some relevant evidence comes from Duke *et al.* (1994), who assessed alcohol comorbidity among 271 people with schizophrenia in South Westminster and found that high levels of alcohol consumption were significantly correlated with severe orofacial tardive dyskinesia. The authors suggest that alcohol use may precipitate tardive dyskinesia in patients taking antipsychotic medications and that this explains the severity of orofacial tardive dyskinesia in patients with highest levels of alcohol use. However, the causal basis of their finding is uncertain, and it would also be possible to explain this finding in terms of individuals with severe tardive dyskinesia or akathisia using alcohol to relieve these unpleasant side effects.

Thus at an individual psychological level of explanation, there is some evidence that people with severe mental illness use drugs to self-medicate negative symptoms, non-psychotic mood problems, anxiety and insomnia. Evidence regarding subjective effects on positive symptoms is less consistent, and the effects of substance use on medication side effects warrant further investigation.

Have changes in the care and social circumstances of people with schizophrenia, particularly deinstitutionalisation, led to a rise in substance misuse in this population?

Other forms of explanation for substance misuse among those with psychotic illnesses focus on the effects of their social environments. Bachrach (1987) has argued that the effects of deinstitutionalisation have led to an increase in the prevalence of dual diagnosis and, further, that living in the community probably does make people with psychotic illness more susceptible to some influences and social trends found in the population as a whole. She describes a generation of 'young adult chronic patients' who have never been institutionalised in long-stay wards but lack adequate social support and activity in the community and have greater access to drugs and alcohol than would have been the case in the asylums. Whether the prevalence of dual diagnosis has in fact increased during the decades during which deinstitutionalisation has been taking place is a question that has been examined by Cuffell (1992). He reviewed published estimates of the prevalence of substance misuse in persons with schizophrenia and found that year of data collection was a very significant variable in explaining variance in reported prevalence rates, with more recently reported studies tending to report higher rates of substance misuse among the severely mentally ill. This is compatible with an increase in the prevalence of dual diagnosis as deinstitutionalisation proceeds; however, no direct causal relationship can be assumed as the rise observed in substance misuse among those with schizophrenia or other psychotic illnesses might simply be a reflection of the increase of substance misuse observed in the general population. For example, illicit drug use in lifetime/ever, past year, and past month epidemiological domains in persons aged 16–29 during the period between 1996 and 1998 all increased at a statistically significant level, with increases in cocaine consumption representing the largest single rise (Home Office 1999). Other studies report that approximately half of those aged 16–22 have ever used an illicit drug, with one study (Boys *et al*. 1999) reporting 98% of young people in the sample using alcohol and 84% using cannabis in the previous 12 months.

Do the social situations and social difficulties of people with schizophrenia lead to substance use?

People with schizophrenia often have problems in finding satisfying activities, relationships and social roles, avoiding boredom and coping with everyday social situations (Lamb 1982). These problems are compounded by the limits on access to ordinary social networks and activities resulting from the stigma attached to mental illness. In a review of the literature, Bergman and Harris (1985) argue that these difficulties are a major factor in the initiation and continuation of drug use in this population, particularly for young people early in the course of their illness. In recent work such as that of the Sainsbury Centre (1998), it is suggested that substance misuse may be one of a constellation of problems experienced by a group of young people with severe mental illnesses who feel alienated from conventional services and society, have never been and see little chance of ever being employed and live in poor and unstable social circumstances. This is the group targeted by assertive outreach services established in the United States and Australia and more recently in the United Kingdom (Sainsbury Centre 1998). A further social difficulty that may be confronted by people with schizophrenia is that they may have fewer skills than others for problem solving and coping with demanding social situations so that drug use becomes a way of coping with situations that otherwise may be distressing and stressful. Lamb (1982) further suggests that difficulties in getting access to a social group can lead those with schizophrenia towards networks of drug users who may be more tolerant and more likely to accept people who are unusual in some way than other social groups. As yet, there is very little evidence available regarding the social contexts in which people with schizophrenia use drugs and alcohol and the ways in which they may find substance use helpful in establishing social networks and coping with demanding social situations and lack of meaningful activity. Further gaps in the available evidence relate to how people with functional psychotic illnesses and the resulting social disabilities negotiate the drug market and obtain substances and how they learn the techniques and regulation of dose levels required by drug use. These questions are particularly pertinent with regard to designing harm minimisation interventions for this group and warrant substantial empirical investigation.

Do people with schizophrenia tend to begin using drugs and alcohol within mental health service settings or in the company of other users of such services?

A further possibility is that drug and alcohol abuse may tend to be disseminated among people with schizophrenia because of wide availability of such substances in mental health service settings, and within social networks of mental health service users. As with other social ways of understanding the basis of dual diagnosis, there is as yet little evidence about the social contexts in which those with schizophrenia are introduced to substance misuse and the sources from which they obtain drugs. In a study of adult in-patients with psychotic illness in London, Phillips and Johnson (2003) found that although a small number of individuals began using substances in mental health service settings (some of whom had commenced use whilse admitted in child or adolescent mental health services), patients who used in the community were very likely to continue such use in hospital (83% used substances on the ward during their current admission). The study also revealed high rates of drug trading among in-patients in the wards sampled for the study.

Previously, in a survey of psychiatric nurses who were members of the UK Royal College of Nursing by Sandford (1995), 68% of respondents were aware of illicit drug use in their workplaces, which were mainly in-patient units. They reported adverse consequences including violence, relapse of illness, drug dealing within wards and mistrust of patients among staff. In a survey carried out in a highly secure forensic hospital by McKeown and

Liebling (1995), reports of cannabis use within the hospital were frequent, with concerns that the persisting supply of drugs to the hospital resulted in increased violence and disruptive behaviour. Evidence is still required about the subcultures within which people with schizophrenia and other functional psychotic illnesses live in the community, the networks which develop between them, and the extent to which people may be introduced to or continue drug use in mental health service settings or with people they have met in mental health service settings.

Conclusion

Currently, the evidence base available to support any explanatory models for substance misuse among those with schizophrenia remains fragmented and limited. At an epidemiological level, there is some evidence in the United States that rates of drug and alcohol abuse among this group do exceed those for the general population, so that it seems appropriate to seek specific explanations for substance misuse in this group. However, this probably does not apply to all substances and has not yet been clearly demonstrated outside the United States. Further, the extent to which this may be explicable in terms of the potentially confounding influence of social deprivation has yet to be established. Reliable evidence regarding the temporal sequence of severe mental illness and substance misuse is difficult to obtain, but so far suggests variations among people with a dual diagnosis in the temporal order in which the two problems arise so that a unitary and generally applicable explanation of the way in which this comorbidity develops is unlikely. At a psychological level, there is fairly robust evidence that substances are used as a form of self-medication, particularly for tension, low mood and anxiety and for negative symptoms, whilse evidence regarding subjective effects on positive symptoms is less clear-cut. Other potential forms of explanation for co-morbid substance misuse relate more to social context than individual psychology, and have as yet probably not received enough consideration, or been investigated enough empirically. Social isolation, boredom, difficulty coping with everyday interactions and lack of meaningful activity all warrant explanation as possible factors in the development of drug and alcohol problems among those with schizophrenia, as do the social networks and social lives of the severely mentally ill and the part substance misuse plays in these.

References

Addington J, Addington D (1998) Effect of substance misuse in early psychosis. *British Journal of Psychiatry* 172 (Supplement 33): 134–136.

Addington J, Duchak V (1997) Reasons for substance use in schizophrenia. *Acta Psychiatrica Scandinavica* 96: 329–333.

Amara S, Sonders M (1998) Neurotransmitter transporters as molecular targets for addictive drugs. *Drug and Alcohol Dependence* 51: 87–96.

Bachrach LL (1987) Leona Bachrach speaks: selected speeches and lectures. *New Directions for Mental Health Services* 35: 1–102.

Baigent M, Holme G, Hafner RJ (1995) Self reports of the interaction between substance abuse and schizophrenia. *Australian and New Zealand Journal of Psychiatry* 29 (1): 69–74.

Bergman HC, Harris M (1985) Substance abuse among young adult chronic patients. *Psychosocial Rehabilitation Journal* 9: 45–54.

Bernadt MW, Murray RM (1986) Psychiatric disorder, drinking and alcoholism: what are the links? *British Journal of Psychiatry* 148: 393–400.

Bidaut-Russell M, Bradford SE, Smith EM (1994) Prevalence of mental illnesses in adult offspring of alcoholic mothers. *Drug and Alcohol Dependence* 35: 81–90.

Boys A, Marsden J, Fountain J, *et al.* (1999) What influences young people's use of drugs? A qualitative study of decision-making. *Drugs: Education, Prevention and Policy* 6 (3): 373–387.

Campbell MS, Moss HB, Daley DC (1993) *Dual Disorders: Counselling Clients with Chemical Dependency and Mental Illness*. Minnesota: Hazelden.

Cantwell R, Brewin J, Glazebrook C, *et al.* (1999) Prevalence of substance misuse in first-episode psychosis. *British Journal of Psychiatry* 174: 150–153.

Caton CLM (1995) Mental service use among homeless and never homeless men with schizophrenia. *Psychiatric Services* 46: 1139–1143.

Cuffell B (1992) Prevalence estimates of substance abuse in schizophrenia and their correlates. *Journal of Nervous and Mental Disease* 180: 589–592.

Dackis CA, Gold MS (1992) Psychiatric hospitals for the treatment of dual diagnosis. In: Lowinson JH, Ruiz P, Millman RB (eds). *Substance Abuse: A Comprehensive Textbook*. Baltimore: Williams and Williams.

Dixon L, Haas G, Wieden P, Sweeney J, Frances A (1990) Acute effects of drug abuse in schizophrenic patients: clinical observations and patients' self-reports. *Schizophrenia Bulletin* 16 (1): 69–79.

Duke PJ, Pantelis C, Barnes TRE (1994) South Westminster Schizophrenia Survey. Alcohol use and its relationship to symptoms, tardive dyskinesia and illness onset. *British Journal of Psychiatry* 164 (5): 630–636.

Fadda F, Rossetti Z (1998) Chronic ethanol consumption: from neuroadaptation to neurodegeneration. *Progress in Neurobiology* 56: 385–431.

Farrell M, Howes S, Taylor C, *et al.* (1998) Substance misuse and psychiatric comorbidity: an overview of the OPCS National Psychiatric Morbidity Survey. *Addictive Behaviours* 23: 909–918.

Hambrecht M, Hafner H (1996) Führen alkohol oder drogenmissbrauch zur schizophrenie? *Nervenarzt* 67: 36–45.

Harrison PJ (1999) The neuropathology of schizophrenia. A critical review of the data and their interpretation. *Brain* 122: 593–624.

Home Office (1999) *Drug Misuse Declared in 1998: Results from the British Crime Survey (Research Study 197)*. London: Home Office.

Johnston LD, O'Malley PM, Evelyn LK (1978) Drugs and delinquency: a search for causal connections. In: Kanel DB (ed). *Longitudinal Research on Drug Use*. Washington DC: Hemisphere.

Khantzian EJ (1985) The self-medication hypothesis of addictive disorders: focus on heroin and cocaine dependence. *American Journal of Psychiatry* 142 (11): 1259–1264.

Kovasznay B, Bromet E, Schwartz JE, Ram R, Lavelle J, Brandon L (1993) Substance abuse and onset of psychotic illness. *Hospital and Community Psychiatry* 44 (6): 567–571.

Lamb HR (1982) Young adult chronic patients: the new drifters. *Hospital and Community Psychiatry* 33 (6): 465–468.

McKeown M, Liebling H (1995) Staff perception of illicit drug use within a special hospital. *Journal of Psychiatric and Mental Health Nursing* 2: 343–350.

Menezes P, Johnson S, Thornicroft G, *et al.* (1996) Drug and alcohol problems among individuals with severe mental illness in South London. *British Journal of Psychiatry* 168: 612–619.

Modestin J, Nussbaumer C, Angst D, Scheidegger P, Hell D (1997) Use of potentially abusive psychotropic substances in psychiatric inpatients. *European Archives of Psychiatry and Clinical Neurosciences* 247: 146–153.

Mueser KT, Drake RE, Wallach MA (1998) Dual diagnosis: a review of etiological theories. *Addictive Behaviours* 23 (6): 717–734.

Mueser KT, Nishith P, Tracy JI, DeGirolamo J, Molinaro M (1995) Expectations and motives for substance use in schizophrenia. *Schizophrenia Bulletin* 21 (3): 367–378.

Nace EP, Davis CW, Gaspari JP (1990) Axis I comorbidity in substance abusers. *American Journal of Psychiatry* 40: 54–56.

Neumann CS, Grimes K, Walker E, Baum K (1995) Developmental pathways to schizophrenia: behavioural subtypes. *Journal of Abnormal Psychology* 104: 558–566.

Noordsy DL, Drake RE, Biesanz JD, McHugo GJ (1994) Family history of alcoholism in schizophrenia. *Journal of Nervous and Mental Disease* 182: 651–655.

Noordsy DL, Drake RE, Teague GB, *et al.* (1991) Subjective experiences related to alcohol use among schizophrenics. *Journal of Nervous and Mental Disease* 179: 410–414.

Phillips P (1998) The mad, the bad and the dangerous – harm reduction in dual diagnosis. *International Journal of Drug Policy* 9: 345–349.

Phillips P, Johnson S (2003) Drug and alcohol misuse among in-patients with psychotic illnesses in three inner London psychiatric units. *Psychiatric Bulletin* 27: 217–220.

Pristach CA, Smith CM (1996) Self reported effects of alcohol use on symptoms of schizophrenia. *Psychiatric Services* 47 (4): 421–423.

Rabinowitz J, Bromet EJ, Lavelle J, Carlson G, Kovasznay B, Schwartz JE (1998) Prevalence and severity of substance use disorder and onset of psychosis in first admission psychotic patients. *Psychological Medicine* 28: 1411–1419.

Regier D, Farmer ME, Rae DS, *et al.* (1990) Comorbidity of mental disorders with alcohol and other drug abuse. *Journal of the American Medical Association* 264 (19): 2511–2518.

Sainsbury Centre for Mental Health (1998) *Keys to Engagement: Review of Care for People with Severe Mental Illness who Are Hard to Engage with Services.* London: Sainsbury Centre.

Sandford T (1995) Drug use is increasing. *Nursing Standard* 9 (38): 16.

Schneier FR, Siris SG (1987) A review of psychoactive substance use and abuse in schizophrenia: patterns of drug choice. *Journal of Nervous and Mental Disease* 175 (11): 641–651.

Serper MR, Alpert M, Trujillo J (1996) Recent cocaine use decreases negative signs in acute schizophrenia: a case study over two consecutive admissions. *Biological Psychiatry* 39: 816–818.

Silver H, Abboud E (1994) Drug abuse in schizophrenia: comparison of patients who began drug abuse before their first admission with those who began abusing drugs after their first admission. *Schizophrenia Research* 13: 57–63.

Soyka M, Albus M, Kathmann N, *et al.* (1993) Prevalence of alcohol and drug abuse in schizophrenic in-patients. *European Archives of Psychiatry and Clinical Neurosciences* 242: 362–372.

Turner WM, Tsuang MT (1990) Impact of substance abuse on the course and outcome of schizophrenia. *Schizophrenia Bulletin* 16 (1): 87–95.

Verdoux H, Mury M, Besanon GM (1996) Etude comparative des conduites toxicomaniaques et les troubles bipolaires, schizophréniques et schizoaffectifs. *L'Encéphale* 22: 95–101.

Chapter 3

Consumer Perspectives

David Webb

Introduction

When we use the language of 'dual diagnosis', and all the other medical terminology that comes with it, such as 'comorbidity', we are participating in the medicalisation of everyday life. Some people call this 'selling sickness' (Moynihan & Cassels 2005) or 'disease mongering' (PLoS 2006). I think it is best described as the medical colonisation of the human spirit. Whatever we call it, we must beware of and resist the excessive medicalising of what it is to be human.

Human experience and medicine

Although almost every aspect of life is being colonised by medicine, nowhere is it perhaps more advanced, and more harmful, than in the mental health industry. In most western societies, the marketing of distressing human experiences as medical conditions is almost complete, with broad community acceptance of the myth that our psychological well-being is determined by the biology of our brains. The notion of 'mental illness' has become so pervasive that this metaphor is now being taken as a literal truth. Not only is the narrow and shallow medical reductionism of modern biological psychiatry causing great harm to individuals caught up in the mental health industry but its blindness to essential aspects of our being also diminishes all of us – our communities, our social fabric and our culture. Mainstream psychiatry today sees only biology so that it not only fails to see that our psyche includes psychology, consciousness and spirituality but also forbids them.

If this sounds exaggerated or alarmist, then consider the current status quo in the mental health industry. If you experience extreme emotional distress that triggers, for instance, suicidal feelings, and you come to the attention of the medical profession then you will almost certainly find yourself with a psychiatric diagnosis, i.e. a medical judgement that you have a mental illness.

We will analyse this a little more closely later, but once this judgment has been made and you have a psychiatric label, your mental illness will almost certainly be treated with psychopharmacological medications. Furthermore, if the doctors also judge that you are incompetent because of your madness, then you will quite likely be forced to take these medications whether you consent to their use or not.

Diagnosis, treatment and human rights

There are three issues we need to look at here – diagnosis, treatment and human rights. But to put this into the context of this book, we need to recognise that this medical way of thinking that has already colonised mental health is now advancing on the drug and alcohol sector under the guise of dual diagnosis. My plea to readers is to resist this colonisation. Indeed, my wish is for the reverse to happen so that some of the knowledge, expertise and wisdom of the drug and alcohol sector can find its way into desperately needed reforms of the mental health industry.

I should perhaps give my 'credentials' to be writing this chapter. My PhD research into suicide, completed in 2006, is relevant to the topic of this book but my primary 'qualification' is that I have experienced both madness and addiction. I was therefore asked to write a 'consumer perspective' on dual diagnosis, so I need to tell a little of my story here. I dread this, however, because it may relegate this chapter – as so often happens with the consumer perspective – to the novelty of the 'human interest' angle that the so-called experts then comment upon. Like many of my colleagues, I assert the exper-tise of the direct, lived experience and reject the tokenistic, 'human interest' role in the discourse around mental health.

Before proceeding, an aside on language is necessary. First, many people around the world, are now (re-)claiming, as I do here, the language of mad-ness in preference to the sterile and stigmatising medical language of mental illness. We do not seek to impose this language on anyone who is not com-fortable with it; but, equally, we do not accept the medical language being imposed on us. Similarly, many of us also reject the label of 'consumer' for similar reasons and prefer to identify as users or ex-users (of psychiatric services) or sometimes as psychiatric survivors. This again is a matter of personal choice and is not to be imposed on anyone by anyone, with my own preference being psychiatric survivor, though I'll use the term 'consumer–survivor' in the rest of this chapter. Now, it's story time …

While in England in 1979, at the age of 24, I spent a few months in a hospital burns unit after an accidental fire following a deliberate overdose. As the years passed, I began to regard it as simply some sort of youthful ab-erration. It was with some surprise then, to say the least, that I found myself suicidal again in 1995. For the next 4 years I struggled with persistent suicidal thoughts, made a couple of serious attempts and several half-hearted, clumsy suicidal 'gestures'. For much of the time, whenever I could, I self-medicated my psychache[1] with heroin.

During the more recent episode, the drug and alcohol services I turned to for help included several short-term (10 days or less) residential 'detox' centres, a couple of longer term (5 weeks to 6 months) residential 'rehab' centres, and various self-help programmes, most notably Alcoholics Anonymous (AA) and Narcotics Anonymous (NA). All of these you could probably call 'psychosocial' (i.e. non-medical/clinical) services. I also did a couple of medicated detoxes in hospital, and the other major medical 'treatment' I received was nearly a year on Methadone. The psychiatric services that I received during this time included two voluntary in-patient admissions to a hospital psychiatric ward (one of less than a week, the other for 3 weeks), and one involuntary admission of only 3 days. I also saw six different psychiatrists over this period, some I saw only once or twice, others for longer (one weekly for about 12 weeks, another for monthly appointments over nearly a year).

Two worlds

From my experience of the two sectors, it is hard to imagine a more stark contrast between ostensibly similar services. Perhaps the most striking contrast occurs when you first walk in through the door. At drug and alcohol services, I was always greeted warmly with a big effort made to try and make me feel as welcome and comfortable as possible. This is especially important the first time you enter a service, which can be intimidating, and you probably do not want to be there at all. Typically this welcome includes one of the 'old-timer' residents (i.e. has been there for more than a few days) showing you around, introducing you to the others, where to get a cup of tea and have a smoke, etc. Sometimes this is formalised into a 'buddy system' as part of the programme. It is a scary thing to step into one of these places, but it helps when you are greeted by someone who has done it themselves just a week or so before you. It also helps that they seem to be doing okay, that maybe you could feel okay soon too.

The psych wards were so very different. First, the admission formalities are cold and clinical as you wait for judgement – like in a courtroom or being dragged before the headmaster – on whether you will be admitted or not. Once you are admitted, you will be shown around, but almost certainly by a nurse or one of the other staff. As you get this tour, you may be introduced

---

[1] A term coined by Professor Edwin S. Shneidman, often regarded as the founding father of (American) suicidology, that he defines as psychological *pain* to distinguish it from the mythical medical illness of 'depression'.

to the other residents, but quite likely not. Social interaction among patients is not facilitated or even encouraged, it seems. It feels like we are expected to be incompetent and incapable of just about anything – otherwise we would not be there, right? And psychiatric wards for me were so unbearably dull and boring that on one occasion I felt I had to leave after about 3 weeks or I would go mad!

Significant contrasts

The drug and alcohol services were mostly active, busy places – even at the detoxes where many of the residents were sick with their withdrawals. Apart from the formal programme of classes, other group activities, homework, etc, there were scheduled walks or other exercise; informal 'meetings' among residents were encouraged, and everybody took part in the cooking and cleaning, generally caring for the space we were living in. If anything, the day was too full of activities so that you sometimes felt you needed some time-out space. Psychiatric wards, in contrast, are characterised by passivity, dullness and boredom. The highlights of the day were meals – trays of hospital food that you had not been involved in the preparation of – and then the drug trolley rounds. There were very few other activities, and the nursing staff always seemed to be busy elsewhere. Watching TV was the main way people killed time before the next meal or the next dose of drugs. Dull, dull, dull – maddeningly dull!

Another striking difference was the make-up of the staff. The staff in drug and alcohol are mostly nonclinical and many, sometimes all of them, are themselves ex-users. Having ex-users on the staff makes for a very different environment. They know what we were going through because they have been there themselves. And we know that. And we know that they know, and they know that we know. And so on. This not only meant that there was an automatic empathy and respect for the hard work of coming off drugs (or booze) but also meant that they knew most of the games we played, with ourselves and with each other, to rationalise or deny our addiction or to think we were somehow different to others in the struggle to get clean/sober. It made for some tough confrontations at times. But it also made for many lively conversations and plenty of laughs, which is another striking difference with sullen, humourless psychiatric wards.

Next, the approach to 'therapy' is very different between the two services, which is highlighted in the language – clinical staff give 'treatment' to patients in psychiatric wards, whereas in drug and alcohol clients or residents are working through their 'recovery' programme. In drug and alcohol, the recovery approach was much more holistic, a whole-of-person approach. Diet, exercise, the busy daily routine of activities, social interactions, conversations, both formal and informal, various responsibilities and duties, such as cooking dinner or being a buddy to a newcomer, etc. were all considered important parts of your recovery programme. In the psychiatric wards, treatment revolved around medication. A couple of times a day the drug trolley would come around, staff would be watching for symptoms and/or side effects and then the doctors would occasionally fine-tune the mix or dosages of the drugs accordingly. That was it.

The final major difference is rarely mentioned in the literature and conferences on dual diagnosis, but it is a critical difference that I wish to highlight in this chapter. Drug and alcohol services are voluntary (unless you're there through a diversion programme of the criminal justice system) whereas at the heart of psychiatric services is the threat of force, of involuntary treatment, a threat that is routinely carried out.

This is inevitably a very shortened version of my story that cannot be taken as either comprehensive or typical. There are many other stories that need to be heard and in much greater detail than the occasional focus group 'snippet' that might find its way into the research literature. The failure of researchers and policy makers to engage meaningfully with the first-person knowledge and expertise of those who know about madness and addiction 'from the inside' is the single greatest weakness in our efforts to develop better policies and services. Furthermore, it is clear that this failing will only be corrected when more researchers and policy makers are themselves consumer–survivors.

Table 3.1 summarises what I regard as the key features that distinguish the two services. What is apparent from this summary is a massive clash of cultures. This culture clash is already recognised and features in current debates around dual diagnosis, though the emphasis tends more to do with differences in institutional infrastructures and the professional status of the workforce rather than in the experience of service users. Instead of

Table 3.1 Service characteristics

Mental health	Drug and alcohol
Medical model	Psychosocial model
Focus on treatment (of illness/symptoms)	Focus on recovery
Biological	More holistic
Pathologises the individual	Considers social context
Emphasises deficits (illness)	Strengths based
Intimidating	Welcoming
Little or no peer support	Strong peer support
Passive participation of patients	Active participation of residents
Mostly clinical staff	Mostly non-clinical staff
Involuntary	Voluntary

addressing each individual item in the table, I want to return to the three key issues of diagnosis, treatment and human rights that underpin the medical colonisation that so concerns me.

Diagnosis

The best that can be said about the scientific status of the current diagnostic system of modern psychiatry is that it is a hypothesis. Some people go further and say that it has as much scientific credibility as astrology, but as a hypothesis it does have some scientific merit. Beyond that, though, the hypothesis that psychological distress is due to some biological malfunction of the brain has not yet been demonstrated (Kutchins & Kirk 1997; Bentall 2004). Despite this, the marketing of the mental illness metaphor, and particularly the 'chemical imbalance of the brain' myth, has been so successful that it has become generally accepted in the community.

Treatment

Given the lack of any solid science behind psychiatry's diagnostic system, it is hardly surprising that the treatments that psychiatry offers for these questionable illnesses also lack scientific credibility. The most severe expression of this is the claim still made by some that psychopharmacological drugs 'fix' the alleged chemical imbalances in the brain. This is not to say that these drugs do not have a role to play, but what they can – and cannot – do needs to be understood (Watkins 2006). Antidepressants, for instance, are best understood as psychological painkillers. The more potent neuroleptic ('antipsychotic') medications are powerful tranquilisers that can sometimes suppress some of the symptoms of so-called psychosis. But these drugs don't 'fix' mental illness any more than morphine fixes broken bones, though it is usually a good idea to have some morphine if you break a leg. Another example of the misleading hype of disease mongering is the current re-packaging of some antipsychotic drugs as 'mood stabilisers' for the sole purpose of expanding the market for these drugs (Healy 2006).

Concern about the excessive medicalisation of madness is sometimes heard even within the mainstream of psychiatry. In 2005, the then President of the American Psychiatric Association, Steven S. Sharfstein, observed that, 'we must examine the fact that as a profession, we have allowed the biopsychosocial model to become the bio-bio-bio model' (Sharfstein 2005). Despite Sharfstein's succinct description of it, the medical colonisation of the psyche marches on, led by his profession.

The third major feature of the mental health industry that distinguishes it from the drug and alcohol sector is the use of force, or 'involuntary treatment', as it is euphemistically called. In most western countries, the use of force is not permitted in drug and alcohol services, in stark contrast to the mental health industry, which has the threat of force at its very foundations, a threat that is carried out daily on thousands of people. Once again, we need to be alert to the misuse of language. One of the slogans of the psychiatric survivor movement is that 'If It's Not Voluntary, It's Not Treatment'. Psychiatric force is about control, not treatment. It is about subduing people, primarily with drugs, in order to control their behaviour, and invariably for the benefit of others around the person rather than for the persons themselves. Medical treatment without consent is not only a violation of a fundamental human rights principle, but it also contradicts, is mutually exclusive with and ultimately self-defeating for any recovery-based service.

There is a clear relationship between medical issues of psychiatric diagnosis and treatment on the one hand and legal issues of the human rights prohibition against medical treatment without consent, on the other. Mental health laws rely on psychiatry to justify depriving a person of the right to refuse treatment. This occurs despite the lack of scientific credibility of psychiatric diagnosis and treatment, which only highlights that psychiatric force is about control, not treatment. There is an urgent need for legal scrutiny of the scientific justification for psychiatric force, but this is a debate for another forum. Meanwhile, these human rights issues will now arise in the drug and alcohol sector as the medical colonisation of the sector proceeds under the guise of 'dual diagnosis'.

Dual diagnosis and policy

This can best be illustrated with a brief description of the current dual diagnosis strategy here in the state of Victoria where I live, followed by a human rights question that exposes a serious flaw in the strategy. A centrepiece of the dual diagnosis strategy here is called the 'No Wrong Door' policy, where the intention is that regardless of which type of service you go to for help, you will get access to the services you need. Central to the No Wrong Door policy is the need for staff from both sectors to be trained to become what is called 'DD aware'. The aim here is not for all staff to also become experts in the other field but to become sufficiently aware to be able to recognise when the other service is necessary and then to make the appropriate referral. The final plank of this policy is to build the relationships between service providers in both sectors so that people are not just given a phone number and sent on their way, falling through the huge cracks as they currently do. The service of the first door walked through takes responsibility for ensuring that the person makes contact with the other service, which may include setting up appointments, personally accompanying them to the other service, or whatever is required. So far so good. Lots of good policy ideas here, though it is still a major challenge to see them implemented.

This policy comes crashing down on the human rights issue of involuntary treatment. And it crashes so badly that it runs the risk of becoming the 'No Right Door' policy. The question I ask policy makers and other leaders in the dual diagnosis debate is

What happens when word gets out on the street that if you go to a drug service for help and they think you're mad, they'll take you up the street to the nuthouse where there's a very good chance they'll lock you up?

So far, I've not received any satisfactory answers to this question. To elaborate this scenario just a little more, we know that the biggest and toughest step to take towards recovery, especially for young people, is the very first step of turning to a service for help. Indeed, one of the greatest challenges in both sectors is how to access those in need of help. We also know that drugs users (and not just illegal drug users) do not like being locked up and, furthermore, that they are extremely skilful at avoiding the lockup. So it would only have to happen a few times before word got out on the street that volunteering yourself to a drug and alcohol service ran the risk of finding yourself locked up in a mental health service. This would be a disaster for drug and alcohol services, especially for young people, with many people avoiding services altogether. The No Wrong Door policy becomes the No Right Door policy.

What can we take from this brief 'consumer perspective' to help us respond better to the needs of those struggling with both madness and addiction? There are three issues I would like to highlight.

First of all, I want to encourage the drug and alcohol sector to stick to their guns and resist the medical colonisation of the sector by psychiatry. The current psychosocial model and recovery-based approach of the sector is the correct approach, not only for drug and alcohol but also for mental health. Indeed, mental health consumers around the world have been calling for psychosocial, recovery-based mental health systems for many years, and although some progress has been made in this direction in some countries, the medical model still remains dominant. Medicine has an important role to play – in both sectors – but the catchphrase that sums up what this role needs to become is 'doctors on tap, not on top'.

Second, the first-person knowledge and expertise of those who know madness and/or addiction 'from the inside' needs to play a much greater role in research, policy and practice – in both sectors. One of the most damaging aspects of medical colonisation is its narrow and shallow third-person perspective (masquerading as 'objectivity') that denies the validity of first-person knowledge. Affirmative action initiatives are required to correct this, such as employment policies to promote greater consumer/survivor participation in the workforce of the services sectors and also in public sector bureaucracies, with special emphasis on creating genuine leadership positions. Likewise, in our universities and research funding bodies, scholarships are needed to bring more of the first-person understanding of madness and/or addiction into the research that will guide policy and practice.

We can look to the achievements of the disability movement over the last 30 years or so to guide us in how to engage more meaningfully with the first-person voice. Under the banner of 'Nothing About Us Without Us', the disability community has asserted the validity and the importance of knowledge grounded in the direct, lived experience of disability. They have also given us the social model of disability, which recognises the social context of disability that is so neglected by the mental health industry and also the drug and alcohol sector, though to a lesser extent. The emergence in recent years of psychosocial disability as part of the social change, human rights disability movement, will have major impact on the mental health industry, which is to be encouraged and supported.

'A safe space to tell our stories' is the phrase that best captures the most critical need for someone facing a crisis of madness and/or addiction. It also highlights the significance of the first-person voice. All healing begins with a story. It may be a story told to a professional therapist or counsellor. It may be a 'sharing' at an AA meeting or some other peer support, self-help group. Or it may simply be confiding in someone close to you. Stories are important. Stories are the primary means for accessing the first-person knowledge of the lived experience, the vital missing 'data' of most current research, policy and practice. Stories and story-telling not only bring out this critical knowledge but also have great healing power. This applies to both the healer and the healed, and there is an urgent need for the healer to heal thyself, which will also require the first-person voice of workers in the field to be heard.

Conclusion

The phrase 'a safe space to tell our stories' also takes us to the final issue I wish to highlight. Whatever spaces we create for people to tell their stories, it is essential that they be a safe space. Force does not work. Human rights principles are important because when they are neglected, harm and suffering inevitably follow. Medical treatment without consent, the cornerstone of the medical colonisation of mental health, automatically creates a very unsafe space. It contradicts and destroys the principles of recovery-based services. Psychosocial healing and psychiatric force cannot coexist. Services for people who experience madness and/or addiction must be motivated by compassion and care rather than the fear and control that motivate most of our mental health systems. We cannot ignore human rights.

References

Bentall RB (2004) *Madness Explained: Psychosis and Human Nature.* London: Penguin.

Healy D (2006) The latest mania: selling bipolar Disorder. *PLoS Medicine* 3 (4), e185 doi:10.1371/journal.pmed.0030185.

Kutchins H, Kirk SA (1997) *Making Us Crazy: DSM – The Psychiatric Bible and the Creation of Mental Disorders.* New York: The Free Press.

Moynihan R, Cassels A (2005) *Selling Sickness: How Drug Companies Are Turning Us All into Patients.* Sydney: Allen & Unwin.

PLoS (2006) A collection of articles from the Inaugural Conference on Disease Mongering April 11–13, 2006, Newcastle, Australia. *PLoS Medicine* 3 (4), http://collections.plos.org/plosmedicine/diseasemongering-2006.php

Sharfstein SS (2005) Big pharma and American psychiatry: the good, the bad, and the ugly. *Psychiatric News* 40 (16): 3.

Watkins J (2006) *Healing Schizophrenia: Using Medication Wisely.* Melbourne: Michelle Anderson Publishing.

Part 2

Common Presentations and Special Populations

Chapter 4

Risk Assessment and Dual Diagnosis

Lisa Reynolds and Jenny Oates

Introduction

Substance misuse is considered to be an indicator of risk for mental health service users. The use of alcohol and illegal drugs by mental health service users has been found to be strongly associated with suicide, self-harm and violence (NICE 2004; Appleby *et al.* 2006). Therefore, risk assessment and management is a priority for individuals who have a dual diagnosis of severe and enduring mental health problems and destabilising substance misuse. Dual diagnosis presents several challenges to the process of risk assessment and management. Individuals with a dual diagnosis are likely to have overlapping and complex needs; thus multiservice involvement is often required. For effective risk assessment and management, care provision must be carefully coordinated and clear systems of communication between services and the service user established. Risk assessment is enhanced when undertaken in partnership with the service user (NIMHE 2004). However, therapeutic engagement of the service user with the risk assessment process may be problematic as service users with dual diagnoses are often viewed negatively by health care professionals (NICE 2004). The challenge for clinicians is to employ a recovery-based approach and assess and manage risk in partnership with the service user.

This chapter will provide a practical guide through the core stages of clinical risk assessment and management. A generic process model for risk assessment will be applied to the needs of service users with a dual diagnosis.

Clinical risk assessment

The Department of Health defines risk assessment and management as

> *... making decisions based on knowledge of the research evidence, knowledge of the individual service user and their social context, knowledge of the service user's own experience, and clinical judgement.* (DH 2007: 7)

The clinician must draw on two main sources of information to guide clinical decisions. Knowledge of statistical factors that have been associated with increased risk is required, together with clinical and contextual information that is specific to the service user's current situation. Evidence of known risk factors may then be sought from the clinical data as well as from the individual's demographic profile. Demographic information, such as the individual's age, gender or past behaviour may be associated with increased risk. However, such factors are static, and thus risk may not be reduced through their modification. Dynamic factors that may be modified, such as those relating to an individual's mental state or socio-economic circumstances, may be more readily used to inform care planning. Thus, contextual information must be gathered in order to situate individuals within their social, cultural and physical environment. Also information specific to the service users including their views, past experiences, and preferences regarding risk management strategies must be incorporated into the risk assessment and management process.

A recovery-based approach to working in partnership with the service user is essential for risk assessment and management, but may also lead to the emergence of tensions and differences of opinion; for example, the *Health Care Commission National Audit on Violence* in mental health services (Royal College of Psychiatrists 2008) has highlighted a disparity between service user and provider perceptions of the association between the use of drugs and alcohol and the incidence of violent behaviour. The commission reported that alcohol was seen as a problem associated with violence by 85% of nurses surveyed, with drugs felt to be a problem by 88% of nurses. In comparison, only 18% of service users felt that alcohol use was a problem and 20% that drug use was a problem in the context of violent behaviour. It is important that any differences in views of risk are identified, discussed and synthesised by both provider and user. Alternative approaches to managing risk might be explored including harm reduction strategies.

Working with the service user to identify their personal relapse signature and develop crisis plans will enable changes in risk status to be responded to both expeditiously and in a sensitive manner. Consideration might be given to working with the service user to create an advance statement to outline how they would wish to be cared for at times of crisis. Working in partnership with the service user to develop advance statements and crisis plans will enable trust to be fostered between service users and providers and is therefore likely to promote early help-seeking behaviour at times of crisis. Risk assessment and management is likely to be affected by delayed engagement with services, with potentially more restrictive risk management measures being employed (Keating & Robertson 2004).

The focus of risk assessment should be to guide and support positive approaches to risk management that will promote engagement with services, social inclusion and thus safe community reintegration (NIMHE 2005). However, when planning care, dilemmas are likely to emerge for the clinician in finding a balance between service user autonomy and the need to ensure public safety. The risk assessment and the risk management plan is where this dilemma must be, at least, acknowledged, if not resolved.

Principles of risk assessment and management

The Department of Health provides (DH 2007) a set of basic principles that underpin risk assessment and management. These are outlined below:

- Risk cannot entirely be eliminated.
- Risk is dynamic and changes over time.
- Risk can be general, specific or both.
- Judgements are not absolutes – our clinical judgement is not the 'final say' on an individual's level of risk.
- Good risk assessment should be undertaken using a team approach.
- Once risk has been identified, it must be managed.

The best practice principles adopted by the Department of Health (2007) remind clinicians to avoid complacency when assessing and managing risk. Remaining vigilant of risk is particularly important when working with dual diagnosis. The National Confidential Inquiry into Homicide and Suicide by People with Mental Illness (Appleby *et al.* 2006) reported that 27% of suicides and 36% of homicides had been committed by service users with a dual diagnosis. The principles also highlight the importance of competent team working. Effective risk assessment and management can only be achieved through the adoption of a coherent, responsive and flexible team approach. Given the complexity of the needs of individuals with dual diagnoses, the coordination and planning of risk assessment and management processes is of vital importance. Team working must include the service user and all agencies involved with the individual's care. Services may share the principles of risk assessment and management but they may have different ways of working, which could prove problematic to synthesise into an integrated risk management plan. For example, on a fundamental level, risk may be conceptualised in many different ways. Individuals and agencies are likely to believe that there is a tacit shared understanding of risk (Dowie 1999). This is evinced by services having differing thresholds for acceptable risk behaviours. In order to avoid misunderstanding, it is important that any risk terminology used is clearly defined and agreed upon by service providers. Agreement should also be reached between service providers regarding the mental health, substance misuse and legal aspects of risk relevant to each individual case.

Service users who have a dual diagnosis have been highlighted as a group who will require the Care Programme Approach (CPA) to ensure the provision of a holistic and coordinated package assessment, support, treatment and care (DH 2008). For CPA, a holistic risk assessment must be undertaken and used to inform a coherent risk management plan. The assessment and management plan must be clearly documented and shared with the service user and all individuals and agencies involved in their care. Consent should be sought from the service user for information to be shared. If information needs to be shared without the service user's consent, the need for confidentiality should be weighed against the assessed risk. The Caldicott principles (DH 1997) and the Data Protection Act 1998 must also be referred to when sharing information.

The process of risk assessment and management

Risk assessment and management is outlined as a stepwise process in the table in Box 4.1. The process is related to dual diagnosis and explored in more depth through the application of the process to a case study.

CASE STUDY 1: JASON

Jason has been admitted to an intensive care ward in an inner city acute mental health unit. He was brought into the 136 suite 2 days ago, and has since been moved to intensive care and placed on section 2 of the Mental Health Act for further assessment. Jason was brought in by police officers who had attended an incident at a local supermarket. Seemingly unprovoked, Jason had shouted at the shopkeeper, threatening to kill him, claiming to have a knife under his jacket. He also made threats to kill the police officers and customers who were in the shop during the incident. However, when Jason was searched he did not have a weapon. The police officers reported that they had observed Jason had told them he was being watched by 'Victor' through their and other people's eyes.

On admission, the ward nursing staff reported that Jason appeared to be paranoid and was responding to auditory hallucinations. He was also very threatening, and smelt of alcohol. Jason admitted drinking several cans of super strength lager and smoking crack cocaine for several days before the incident. Since admission, Jason has only provided minimal personal details. He has given a name and a date of birth and told the assessing doctor that he had travelled from Manchester to London a week ago to visit his brother Mark. When asked about his brother, Mark, Jason has said, 'if I see him I'll kill him. Don't bring that **** anywhere near me.'

Since admission, Jason has tried to leave the ward five times. He has been aggressive towards other service users and ward staff. He has also made threats to kill the staff who have prevented him from leaving the ward.

Box 4.1 The process of risk assessment and management

Context
Situate the assessment within a specific social context or environment, for example, community or ward setting. Is the context time limited?

Defining the risks
Do you need to undertake a global risk assessment or are you concerned about specific risks, for example, of suicide or self-harm?

Identifying who is at risk
Consider who might be harmed and how; is there an identified potential victim?

Information gathering
Try to use several sources of information in order to capture different perspectives of the risk presented by or to the service user.

Evaluating the risks
Compare the information gathered against the current research evidence base (e.g. statistical risk factors). Information must be considered a specific environmental or social context and ideally be undertaken in partnership with the service user. Consider whether any additional information is required to make the assessment more robust.

Deciding which risk factors can be modified
Identify which factors might be changed to decrease the assessed risk.

Resource implications
Decide what resources are needed and which agencies need to be involved to modify the risk factors that have been identified.

Communication
Record the findings of the assessment and disseminate information about assessed risk.

Care planning
Plan care in partnership with the service user to contain and reduce the risks identified.

Review
Set a review date for the assessment and care plan. Risk assessment should also be updated if the service user's situation or presentation changes significantly.

Step 1:   *Situating the assessment within the social and environmental context*

Risk assessment must be related to specific conditions or situations, for example, whether the service user is in a ward or a community setting. Jason has been taken from the community by the police to an acute mental health unit as a place of safety. The risk assessment must include information regarding the ward environment. As Jason presents a risk of absconsion and violence, this might include the physical and procedural levels of security that the ward affords.

The promotion of a safe ward environment requires good communication and team working, and a constant awareness of service user whereabouts and activity. Potential hazards may be temporal and relate to specific times of day, for example, mealtimes and meeting times when there is more activity on the ward. Jason has also made several attempts to leave the ward, and this is a source of aggravation for him. Ward staff must identify the conflict around leaving the ward as a hazard point for Jason and determine a management plan that maintains staff and patient safety every time he attempts to leave. It may be more proactive to spend more time with Jason explaining his detention and working with him to avoid repeated conflict about this issue.

Step 2:   *Defining the risks*

Risks may be broadly categorised into risks to self and others. Risks of suicide, self-harm, self-neglect, violence and offending must be considered alongside risks directly related to substance misuse. Risks to dependents of the service user, in particular, children, must also be assessed. If a risk to dependants is identified, then referral should be made to relevant agencies such as Safeguarding Children teams so that a more specialised assessment can be undertaken.

Jason presents a clear risk of violence, because he is making threats towards specific individuals. His apparent fear of 'Victor' and anger with his brother denote that he considers himself to be at risk from others. Therefore he might become violent in order to defend himself against perceived threats. He could also potentially be a risk of harm to himself. Therapeutic engagement is vital here. Staff need to know if Jason develops suicidal ideas or thoughts of violence. This information is only going to come from talking with him, and getting his perspective on the potential risks he faces and poses.

Ward staff must be vigilant regarding the potential after-effects of Jason's alcohol and crack use. He may experience symptoms of acute alcohol withdrawal and crack withdrawal. These may include severe low mood and potential suicidal ideation, particularly when twinned with his present paranoia. While use of alcohol and cocaine may increase risky behaviour because of their disinhibiting effects, withdrawal brings its own risks. In Jason's case, we can see two of the three main ways in which substance use corresponds to an increase in potential risk: first, the increase in emotional volatility that some substances, particularly alcohol and stimulants, may engender; and secondly, the rapid decline in mood and ability to cope that withdrawal from these substances brings. The third way in which substances may interact with risk – the deleterious effect of perpetual or habitual substance misuse on mental state, motivation and social circumstances – may also be a factor here. This may become evident, once more is known about Jason's personal history.

Step 3:   *Identifying who is at risk*

Jason presents both a generalised and specific risk to others. In the acute ward environment, there is a general risk of violence from Jason towards all staff and patients because of his belief that he is being watched by 'Victor' through them. There is also a possible risk to self.

Jason has made threats to kill his brother. Therefore, a potential victim of his violent behaviour has been identified.

Step 4:   *Information gathering*

Risk assessment involves bringing together a comprehensive collection of information, evidence from research epidemiology and clinical practice. Clinicians have access to a wide range of sources of information. These include interviews with the service user, carers and relatives and reports and documentation related to service users' previous contact with health or social services and police or prison records. It is unlikely that all sources of information will be available at the service user's point of contact with health care services; therefore it is important to record what information is missing, to make a judgement as to how the missing information might affect the outcome of the initial assessment and to consider including further information gathering within the plan of care that is subsequently devised.

The team must endeavour to get more information from Jason about his background. Information from Jason's GP, his prison details and his previous contact with health and social services would enable the team to appreciate the history and context of this current presentation and would make a thorough risk assessment possible. Contact with Jason's brother or another relative who may have an insight into his history and current concerns would also be beneficial here.

If Jason continues to be unforthcoming about his history, ward staff may need to do detective work: ringing accident and emergency departments and community mental health teams (CMHTs) in his area of origin or requesting information from local prisons. Jason's collaboration is dependent upon him being engaged in this risk assessment process.

When tracing Jason's history, the team should also consider his contact with non-statutory agencies. He may be known to drug and alcohol services in prison or in the voluntary sector. In either case, these services may not immediately share information with the ward. Clear relevant information sharing is more likely if the team can make a written request stating the concerns that have led to risk assessment and why the information sought is vital to completing the risk assessment and management process.

Step 5:   *Evaluate and formulate risks from a service user and a service provider perspective*

Many global and specific risk assessment tools are available to help structure and inform clinical evaluation of risk. Consideration must be given to choosing a risk assessment tool that will enable risks relating to the client group to be assessed and will be practical given the time available and the system of multidisciplinary team (MDT) functioning. It is important that the approach taken to risk assessment is adapted to the needs of the service user group concerned. For service users with a dual diagnosis, specific substance misuse-related risks must also be considered when undertaking an assessment.

Jason's presentation is a typical profile of someone at high risk of harming himself or others. He is a young man, recently released from prison, using illicit drugs, presenting as a psychotic, apparently homeless and lacking social supports. This profile, based on what we know statistically about high-risk individuals is only half of the picture and will need to be considered from Jason's perspective. Eliciting Jason's views of risk can provide ward staff with a means of working with him, by identifying his concerns and developing a shared approach to their management.

From a service perspective, the formulation of risk may be that Jason presents an imminent risk to others. He is known to services elsewhere and should probably be transferred to those services – perhaps to a psychiatric intensive care unit (PICU) setting, depending on what information is gathered about his past and current care. His current fears may have some basis in real events and he may well be under threat from his associates. Recent crack use and a come down from this binge also appear to be factors in his presentation. Jason is also in a high-risk group for suicide and homicide – a young man with no social supports and a forensic history.

Jason's evaluation of his situation is 'I'm under threat from "Victor". I'm in hospital but I don't feel safe here. I don't feel safe to contact family, and I don't want to go back to the services I've used in the past'.

There is a clear difference in priorities here, between the clinical and service user's formulation of risk. Jason is focused on risk from others, whereas a service perspective on risk would be focused on risks he poses to others, and potentially, to himself.

Step 6:   *Clinical risk management: which factors can be modified?*

The ward team must determine which of the risk factors arising from the assessment may be modified using available resources. Individual practitioners must also be aware of their attitudes and beliefs and consider how these might impact upon how they engage with the service user in managing identified risks (Royal College of Psychiatrists 2008).

Admission to hospital has modified some of the risks for Jason as he is being observed closely and prevented from accessing illicit drugs. He also has access to food and shelter and psychiatric care. While supporting Jason through close observation, the ward team should not just be preventing him from harming others through removal of opportunities to harm. Effective risk management uses the formulation of risk to identify modifiable factors. Jason feels under threat. Is there any way that staff can help decrease his anxiety about 'Victor' or about being watched? Jason does not want family contact. Can we negotiate with him to allow us to contact another person he does trust at this time? Are there any ways we can encourage Jason to trust the ward team?

This admission is not just about creating a safe environment for Jason. It is also an opportunity to review and begin to address the reasons why Jason presents as such a high risk: his lack of social support, his psychotic symptoms and his drug and alcohol use. The risk management plan should include consideration of what social support Jason may benefit from on discharge and who should provide him with that support. A debate may ensue about who should provide after-care for Jason, particularly if he is out of area, but once factors relating to his home situation have been identified in his risk assessment, the team is duty bound to address them in his management plan. A degree of realism about Jason's motivation regarding altering his drug use would be beneficial here.

Step 7:   *Determining what resources are needed*

Determining what resources are required and who should be involved in Jason's care will depend on the information gathered in Jason's assessment. Jason may have been in the care of his prison CMHT or drugs services and may well have been referred to local services before release. If no services are currently working with him, the ward team have the opportunity to consider what approach Jason is most likely to respond to. It might be worth exploring whether the local CMHT has a dual diagnosis specialist, or if local services work closely with non-statutory drug agencies. The team will also need to know whether statutory drug services will work with service users who have a forensic history. It is important to ascertain what has worked or not worked for Jason in the past and whether Jason will tolerate a multi-agency approach, or if he is most likely to engage with a single agency and a single key worker.

In the context of risk management, the team's objectives are to match services to Jason's needs. Multi-agency management of risk depends on clear communication, information sharing and a clear understanding of roles and responsibilities. Jason has been admitted to hospital with no obvious support network, which suggests that he finds maintaining relationships difficult. He has not made the transition from one institution (prison) to the community successfully and has been quickly admitted to a second institution. Effective matching of resources to the individual requires Jason to be involved in making referral decisions.

Step 8:   *Communication*

The complexities of risk are often difficult to communicate. Communication via documentation may take the form of an initial risk assessment and management plan, and of a more detailed comprehensive assessment, as information is gathered. Key information to be documented and communicated includes the nature or type of risk, the severity and likelihood of that risk, the time frame for the risk, whether the risk is imminent, immediate or time limited and finally who is at risk.

If Jason is to be referred to other services then the risk assessment needs to be concise and comprehensive in a format that makes sense to other services. Sharing of risk information is a vital element of referring to other services, and of the CPA. When formulations of risk are shared with other services, it is vital that there is a shared terminology and appreciation of risk, along with a shared consideration of how that information will be used. The Caldicott principles (DH 1997) should guide any decisions on who to provide information to, in what format or level and how they will use it. As with all risk assessments, the ward team need to consider sharing the information they share with others with Jason and to advise him of how this information is to be used. If the risk assessment is not to be shared with Jason at this time, then the reasoning behind this decision should be documented.

Step 9:   *Care planning*

In considering Jason's risks, it has become clear that he has short-term and long-term needs, and that a comprehensive risk management should incorporate planning for the future as well as direct immediate care. We may differentiate between these by considering ward-based care planning, on the one hand, and CPA care planning, on the other.

As Jason's clinical presentation alters, so will his dual diagnosis needs and the level of risk presented. Planning for Jason's long-term needs must begin with an appreciation of his perspective on care provision. Does he want to stop hearing voices and to have social support? If so, then this is the starting point for therapeutic work, alongside the prevention of risk behaviour and maintenance of Jason's safety.

As risk information is shared, and referrals to other services are made, the CPA guides process and procedure. Calling a CPA meeting early in admission can enable all involved to have clear notions of their roles and responsibilities with regard to risk management. The CPA meeting is also an opportunity for all involved to discuss and clarify the meaning and importance of risks. Differences of interpretation and priorities can be resolved or acknowledged here. Within a CPA care plan there should be scope to identify appropriate therapeutic interventions, such as motivational interviewing or harm reduction strategies. The plan should also acknowledge Jason's early warning signs, relapse signature and crisis and contingency plans.

Step 10:   *Set a review date for assessment and care plan*

Reviewing and updating risk assessments and care plans should occur routinely and as circumstances change. In Jason's case, his risks will change as his presentation changes and as he changes environments, for example, from a secure to an open ward, and from hospital to the community. Regular review should occur so that the success and appropriateness of Jason's involvement with services is monitored and acknowledged.

Conclusion

The complexities of risk are greatly simplified by clinical risk assessment tools and procedures. However, for effective risk assessment and management, a complete picture must be built of the individual and potential risks posed. Risk can never be entirely eliminated, and clinicians need to remain mindful of risk even after systems of management have been put in place. It is important that the causes of incidents are analysed and lessons learnt. Safety issues need to be openly discussed and near misses and errors reflected upon by all individuals involved in the provision of care (Weick & Sutcliffe 2007). However, tensions often exist between organisational measures of performance and the reality of working with the complexities of risk and recovery. It is important that an open culture in which concerns about risk may be safely shared is cultivated through regular training, supervision and effective leadership. Services need to support the process of risk assessment and management through the use of non-blame systems for reporting incidents and promoting organisational learning.

References

Appleby L, Shaw J, Kapur N, *et al.* (2006) Avoidable deaths: five year report by the National Confidential Inquiry into Suicide and Homicide by People with Mental Illness. www.medicine.manchester.ac.uk/suicideprevention/nci/Inquiry_publications/inquiry_publications_2006 (accessed 4.8.08).

Department of Health (1997) *The Caldicott Committee. Report on the Review of Patient-Identifiable Information.* London: DH.

Department of Health (2007) *Best Practice in Managing Risk: Principles and Guidance for Best Practice in Managing Risk to Self and Others in Mental Health Services.* London: DH.

Department of Health (2008) *Refocusing the Care Programme Approach.* London: DH.

Dowie J (1999) Communication for better decisions: not about risk. *Health Risk and Society* 1 (1): 41–53.

Keating F, Robertson D (2004) Fear, black people and mental illness: a vicious circle? *Health and Social Care in the Community* 12 (5): 439–447.

National Institute of Clinical Excellence (NICE) (2004) Self-harm: the short-term physical and psychological management and secondary prevention of self-harm in primary and secondary care. http://www.nice.org.uk/guidance/index.jsp?action=download&o=29424 (accessed 4.8.08).

National Institute for Mental Health in England (NIMHE) (2004) *The Ten Essential Shared Capabilities – A Framework for the Whole of the Mental Health Workforce*. London: NIMHE.

National Institute for Mental Health in England (NIMHE) (2005) *NIMHE Guiding Statement on Recovery*. London: NIMHE.

Royal College of Psychiatrists (2008) Health Care Commission National Audit of Violence 2006–2007. Final report – working age adult services. http://www.rcpsych.ac.uk/PDF/!removed-WAA%20Nat%20Report%20final%20for%20Leads%2010%2012.pdf (accessed 5.8.08).

Weick KE, Sutcliffe KM (2007) *Managing the Unexpected. Resilient Performance in an Age of Uncertainty*. San Francisco, CA: John Wiley and Sons.

Chapter 5

Reducing Drug-Related Harm Among Mentally Ill People

Peter Phillips

Introduction

There are a host of reasons why dual diagnosis has emerged as a significant clinical issue during the past decade, both in the United Kingdom and internationally. There is equivocal evidence that there are increased rates of violence and offending among this group, higher rates of homelessness (when compared to those with either single diagnosis), a greater array of pressing social needs and physical health problems (including higher rates of blood-borne viral illnesses such as HIV and hepatitis C), higher rates of suicide, higher service costs, and major difficulties in engaging and retaining those with a dual diagnosis in formal service contact (let alone traditional drug treatment programmes) (Cuffell 1992; Smith & Hucker 1994; Phillips & Labrow 1998; Phillips & Johnson 2001).

Interventions and approaches

Given these concerns, it seems critical to use evidence-based approaches for the care and management of individuals with this combination of problems in order to engage them in interventions or treatments with known efficacy. As is stated elsewhere in this text (Chapter 22) at the current time such interventions remain elusive, and it is unlikely that a single, designed treatment approach would ever be broad enough to encompass the heterogeneity of individuals presenting with dual diagnosis. Added to this picture is the rigid adoption of traditional treatment approaches to substance use (abstinence and recovery models) by traditional mental health services. While abstinence may be a laudable final goal for these individuals, it may not be realistic or practical in the first instance to consider it as a clinical goal for all individuals presenting in mental health service settings. Promoting such changes while individuals are acutely unwell, with high stress levels, is unlikely to lead to lasting change. For example, attempting to make changes to substance use behaviours while the individual is actively psychotic and paranoid may not be effective. This leaves a gap for clinicians who want to be able to offer some form of effective help. Withholding care or treatment is generally not an option, often because of the fact that many individuals with dual diagnosis are detained under mental health legislation (Phillips 1998; Phillips & Johnson 2003).

Harm reduction

Harm reduction approaches to substance use and misuse began in the Netherlands (where drug policy is based on public health and socio-medical approaches) and were led by organisations like the junkiebond and in the United Kingdom in the early 1980s, primarily as a response to human immunodeficiency virus (HIV) and concern about widespread transmission of the virus in the heterosexual community through the partners of intravenous drug users. This was summed up by the (United Kingdom) Advisory Committee on the Misuse of Drugs (ACMD), which suggested that the risk to public health from HIV was greater than that posed by drug misuse. In the United Kingdom, harm reduction was initially focused then on drug use through injection (particularly heroin). Needle and syringe exchange programmes were established, and a low threshold approach was adopted as a service model. Since that time, harm reduction has continued to cause controversy, being adopted as government policy in much of Europe and the developing world, while at the same time harm reduction programmes are legally prevented from accessing state funds in other countries (e.g. United States).

There is no single definition of harm reduction (a term used interchangeably with harm minimisation), but Lenton and Single (1998) have suggested the following:

- The primary goal is the reduction of drug-related harms rather than drug use per se.
- Interventions or strategies are included for individuals who continue to use (in order to maximise safety in use).
- Strategies are used that demonstrate whether the overall strategy is likely to result in net reduction of drug-related harms.

Riley and O'Hare (2000) have defined harm reduction as having several main characteristics: *pragmatism* (accepting that substance use exists, and rather than ignoring, condemning or criminalising individuals who use substances, we should work towards minimising its harmful effects, acknowledging that some ways of using drugs are safer than others), *humanistic values* (avoiding moralistic judgements about drug use and supporting the dignity of the user), *focus on harms* (whether an individual uses or not is important, but harms to individual and community health and social and economic functioning are the focus. The priority is to reduce harms of drug use to users and others, not necessarily drug use itself) and *environment* (acknowledging poverty, social class, racism, social isolation, gender discrimination and inequalities affect vulnerability to and capacity for managing substance-related harms).

These ways of defining harm reduction clearly locate it as a public health-orientated intervention, which addresses the practicalities of substance use in the present and focuses on the actual and tangible reduction of drug-related harms as the priority.

Using harm reduction approaches with mentally ill individuals

Much has been written about the efficacy of harm reduction approaches with populations of (injecting) drug users, but at the current time there is little research that evaluates the efficacy of such approaches with the mentally ill. Despite this, a number of practical guides have been established, based on the combination of a range of psychosocial and psychological interventions with harm reduction approaches. This has been described particularly well by Carey (1996) who discusses the use of harm reduction interventions as part of a package of collaborative, motivation-based approaches to substance use reduction among the mentally ill.

Carey's (1996) approach blends psychosocial interventions with elements of assertive community treatment to produce a five-stage management and intervention model that uses the transtheoretical model of change (Prochaska & DiClemente 1982) (discussed by Callaghan in Chapter 7) as a basis for understanding how individuals make changes to their substance use behaviours (stages of change) and blends this with the matching severity of illness to intensity of service contact, emphasising social functioning, motivational interviewing (using cognitive dissonance) and harm reduction in a five-stage intervention model for working with mentally ill substance users.

Carey notes that harm reduction approaches provide an alternative to abstinence-only programmes, and therefore are more likely to have impact for those patients who have not considered a drug-free life as a goal. Often those using mental health services do not approach services for help with their drug use, and such intervention may not be welcome.

The approach is sometimes described as 'meeting users where they are at, with no hard and fast rules', and is based on the construct that substance use occurs on a continuum of use, ranging from abstinence to harmful use/dependence. This notion or way of working accepts that if an individual reduces the quantity of a substance used or the frequency of its use, then adverse consequences (harms) are also likely to be reduced. Further, there are clearly more harmful, and 'safer' or less harmful ways of using any substance. For example, at a basic level, regularly substituting a fruit juice or soda for an alcoholic drink reduces the overall consumption of alcohol in a drinking session; and sniffing or chasing heroin is less harmful (and less potentially dangerous for overdose) than injecting the drug. Movements along the continuum of use are to be encouraged, rather than choosing to emphasise that a client is not yet completely drug free.

CASE STUDY 1

Michael is 34 and has been living with schizophrenia for the last 15 years. He lives in a supported hostel for the mentally ill, but is regularly admitted to the psychiatric hospital (on average two or three times each year) during periods when his illness is exacerbated, and he is unable to cope. He has a good relationship with his CPN (community mental health nurse) and has limited contact with his family (his mother [Mildred] is elderly and lives with his other brother). Michael's mother has always believed that cannabis use was the reason Michael developed schizophrenia in the first place and tends to raise these views with Michael when things are starting to deteriorate.

Michael usually smokes less than five joints on most days (often three to four), and typically smokes with two friends in the evening (one from the hostel and another who lives locally). They tend to smoke at the friend's flat or in the small park opposite the local pub. Michael's cannabis use began to increase after his mother was hospitalised when she became very unwell with pneumonia. Mildred started to express her worries about his illness, and in her view, he had 'brought it on himself' and was 'making it worse everyday by smoking more of the stuff'. Michael's brother Pete finds the conflict over his brother's cannabis use amusing and tends to make fun of the situation (which distresses his mother further). Michael's cannabis use doubles over the course of a week, and the circumstances of his use change (he begins smoking in his room in the hostel, soon after he wakes up in the morning – he finds that this distracts him from ruminating about his mother's illness and criticism of his use). Hostel staff quickly pick up that he is using cannabis in the hostel premises (the smell), and he is formally warned about use and threatened with eviction if use continues (this contributes to Michael's paranoia and becomes the subject of his auditory hallucinations). Michael tries to contact his CPN after his mother's condition deteriorates and the hospital contacts Michael to attend, but discovers his CPN is not at work because of illness (a locum is covering and offers to see Michael at the team base). These events lead to further cannabis (and alcohol) use, and when Michael returns to the hostel he is reprimanded by staff (as he appears intoxicated). The next day Michael is guarded, suspicious, constantly responding to voices and appears angry and irritable. The hostel manager arranges admission to the psychiatric hospital and later the same day Michael is admitted (informally).

Responses to the case study

Michael's response to his circumstances is not unusual in the context of schizophrenic illness. His relationship with his mother is characterised by criticism and blaming, and at a time of extreme stress his cannabis use increases (as a means of coping with stress and increased symptoms). It should be noted that Michael's regular use of cannabis is a well-established part of his social life that does not seem to cause adverse consequences.

In this sense, the harms from Michael's drug use have come not from using cannabis, but from using it outside his 'regular' pattern (i.e. more frequently and in higher volume). Further, regular use of cannabis is a social activity and therefore 'joints' are shared and conversation held. Therefore use during this episode has the potential for exacerbating Michael's paranoid symptoms and making him feel more guarded and suspicious.

Using harm reduction approaches with Michael

The aim of using harm reduction approaches with individuals in Michael's situation is not to get them to completely stop using, as discussed earlier, but to make their use as safe as possible. Verbalising this to Michael may have a powerful effect and should facilitate open and honest dialogue about his use of cannabis.

Although Michael is aware that others believe his cannabis use has exacerbated his mental illness, he clearly does not accept this, and continues to regularly enjoy smoking cannabis with his friends. In this regard, he is 'pre-contemplative' and interventions should be based around raising his concern over his drug use. The CPN should try to elicit these concerns from Michael himself. This might be undertaken by helping Michael to link his increased symptoms and difficulties at the hostel with his increased cannabis use (e.g. using a diary approach detailing use per day). This should be undertaken in an exploratory and collaborative manner and should not involve use of confrontative or prescriptive interventions.

Good mental health care provision would also involve addressing the concerns of the hostel staff with Michael, and it may be that Michael makes agreements with staff about the use of hostel facilities when he appears intoxicated or 'high' to others.

This is not an exhaustive list of interventions, but rather an indication of the types of approaches and interventions that might be used in a harm reduction framework. What would be used, and how, would depend on the individual circumstances and the therapeutic relationship between Michael and the mental health and social care workers involved in his care.

Dual diagnosis and harm reduction: the future?

If we are to consider a more pragmatic and realistic approach to working with those with a dual diagnosis, there are a number of questions that must be answered in order to develop effective and responsive harm reduction strategies, which are acceptable and appropriate to the communities with whom they are developed. These questions concern how drug types are selected, how dose is established, how using limits are self-imposed or imposed by others, how reliable sources of information are accessed (such as experienced users) and how the drug market is negotiated by those with sometimes profound social disability. Other pertinent questions concern the role of user and peer networks among those with a dual diagnosis, since it is well recognised that these networks are integral to the construction and dissemination of drug-using practices. Solutions to these questions should facilitate a collaborative and effective approach, which encompasses both public and mental health paradigms.

Conclusion

The evidence about the role of drugs in the development of mental illness is not consistent, and debate still continues about whether drug use can itself lead to the development of long-term psychotic illness. However, despite these concerns there are a large number of clear advantages of utilising harm reduction approaches to those with a dual diagnosis. Both experience and the literature are clear regarding the effectiveness of harm reduction with other groups of drug users. It is also clear that using harm reduction approaches impacts positively on service engagement and retention rates because services and goals are individually tailored to the individual needs and realities of the client, accepting them as and where they are, with no hard and fast rules. Crucially, in the dual diagnosis context harm reduction may also be about accepting that drug use may have benefits as well as disadvantages for individuals.

In summary, to start to address the inadequacy of service provision and intervention for those with mental health problems and problematic substance use, services should adopt appropriate harm reduction strategies into their clinical programmes and staff training as part of a recognition that insisting on abstinence often means 'you'll never see them again'.

References

Carey KB (1996) Substance use reduction in the context of outpatient psychiatric treatment: a collaborative, motivational, harm reduction approach. *Community Mental Health Journal* 32 (3): 291–306.

Cuffell B (1992) Prevalence estimates of substance abuse in schizophrenia and their correlates. *Journal of Nervous and Mental Disease* 180: 589.

Lenton S, Single E (1998) The definition of harm reduction. *Drug and Alcohol Review* 17 (2): 213–219.

Phillips P (1998) The mad, the bad and the dangerous – harm reduction in dual diagnosis. *International Journal of Drug Policy* 9 (5): 345–349.

Phillips P, Johnson S (2001) How do drug and alcohol misuse develop among the severely mentally ill? A literature review. *Social Psychiatry and Psychiatric Epidemiology* 36: 269–276.

Phillips P, Johnson S (2003) Drug and alcohol use among in-patients in three inner London psychiatric units. *Psychiatric Bulletin* 27: 217–220.

Phillips P, Labrow J (1998) *Understanding Dual Diagnosis*. London: MIND Publications.

Prochaska JO, DiClemente C (1982) Transtheoretical therapy: toward a more integrative model of change. *Psychotherapy: Theory, Research and Practice* 19 (3): 276–288.

Riley D, O'Hare P (2000) Harm reduction: history, definition and practice. In: Inciardi JA, Harrison LD (eds). *Harm Reduction: National and International Perspectives*. Thousand Oaks, CA: SAGE.

Smith J, Hucker S (1994) Schizophrenia and substance abuse. *British Journal of Psychiatry* 165: 13–21.

Chapter 6

Motivational Interviewing

Chris Glover

Introduction

Health workers routinely describe people presenting with dual diagnosis as 'challenging to work with'. Mental health and drug workers may benefit from training in motivational interviewing (MI) as it may help them develop a greater sense of the complexity of behaviour change and adopt more realistic goal setting with clients, which in turn helps preserve the therapeutic relationship and maximises the potential for success in future attempts at behaviour change.

Motivational interviewing is an evidence-based way of working with people in order to enable them to make changes in their lives. The evidence to date is largely concerned with reduction or cessation of substance use (Noonan & Moyers 1997), but in recent years there is much to support other behaviours related to health (Resnicow *et al.* 2001). While at present the evidence to support its application with coexisting disorders is less strong, the focus of this chapter is to suggest that training mental health staff in MI principles and techniques enables them to develop a good relationship with the client and establish more realistic, achievable goals. If the plan is not achieved at that point (substance misuse being a chronic relapsing condition) with many attempts at change required before permanent change is achieved, what both worker and patient are left with is a faulty plan, rather than a faulty patient or worker. The relationship can remain intact. This may appear to some as rather negative, but it is not about expecting failure; it is concerned with a realistic approach in order to preserve a therapeutic relationship, and as a result, continued work in the future.

What is MI?

The background to MI is the cycle of change (Prochaska & DiClemente 1984). This describes change as being a six-part process with which many readers will be familiar (Figure 6.1).

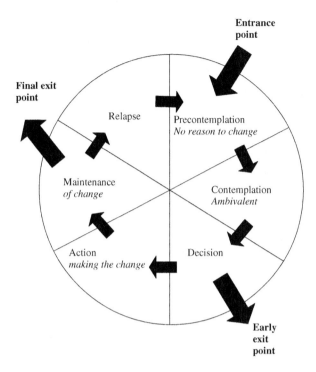

Figure 6.1 The 'Stages of Change' model. Reproduced from Prochaska and DiClemente (1984) with permission.

In phase one, a person is precontemplative, not wishing at all to make any changes to their behaviour. This group is perhaps the largest group found in those with coexisting disorders, and, therefore, the largest group mental health staff will be working with. Rather than working towards reduction or abstinence at this point, staff need to attempt to raise the person's awareness of the use of a substance in relation to the current situation.

Some small or large, external or internal influence may make the precontemplative person consider change to his or her behaviour, making him or her contemplative. The role of the worker at this point is to try and enable the client to resolve ambivalence.

Provided some ambivalence is resolved (but it is never far away), the client moves into the next phase of preparation, where he or she is committed to and planning to make change, and here the worker can help pinpoint how he or she may go about this.

Action is the next phase with the client making changes as planned.

If all goes well, the client moves into the next phase, maintenance, with the worker helping him or her to develop new skills in order to adapt to a reduced use, or abstinent lifestyle.

The cycle can be exited at any point. At this point, however, the client either manages to maintain the planned changes or may experience a lapse or relapse. The first is a short-lived resumption of the previous behaviour or use, the latter a full-blown resumption of the previous behaviour.

Motivational interviewing is based upon the following four general principles (Miller & Rollnick 2002):

- Express empathy
- Develop discrepancy
- Roll with resistance
- Support self-efficacy

Expressing empathy: This is of course a principle that is necessary with any form of counselling style or technique. We know from evidence (Project MATCH Research Group 1997) that forming a good relationship with a client is the largest factor affecting the outcome of any treatment, and a client experiencing a worker as being empathic towards him or her is part of developing a good working relationship.

Developing discrepancy: This is perhaps more specifically linked to MI than other approaches to treatment. As workers, we are trying to help clients resolve the ambivalence they feel about altering their behaviour, wanting on the one hand to make changes and on the other for things to stay exactly as they are, without the complications that their substance use brings to their lives. Developing discrepancy can be a very tricky area when working with clients, as it is concerned with bringing the client's attention to those parts of their current behaviour that do not fit with their own important personal goals and beliefs. Put baldly, no client ever thought to themselves as a child 'I want to be a crack user when I grow up'. In order to develop a client's discrepancy, it is important to tease out from that individual exactly what their own personal goals and values are, as they will be different for each individual, and examine how these boundaries may be, being crossed as a result of the client's current behaviour. This needs to be achieved carefully, with no sense of judgement on the part of the worker.

Roll with resistance: Many forms of treatment for substance misuse utilise confrontation as a means of dealing with some of the denial associated with long-term damage and use. Many of these approaches are extremely successful with clients. The exception is when a client is suffering from a severe mental illness where such confrontation may well lead to psychotic decompensation and relapse, because of exposure to high levels of expressed emotion. However, MI does not use this approach. If resistance is encountered with a client, there are a variety of different methods, such as altering the plan for change or reflecting back on what the client is saying. Resistance is never directly opposed, and the worker never argues for change with the client.

Supporting self-efficacy: Here the worker needs to convey to the client that the client's own belief in their ability to make changes is supported wholeheartedly by the worker. Clinically, this is not always easy.

There are four main opening strategies, which are as follows (Miller & Rollnick 2002):

Open-ended questions
This strategy will be familiar to all workers, whatever approach they may be using. An open question is one that does not elicit a yes or no answer. We are trying to find out as much as we can from the client. When using the MI approach, we will be particularly concerned with remembering what the client has said, in the same words where possible.

Affirming
It is important for workers to acknowledge achievements by clients verbally, and it could be argued that this does not happen as often as it might. Clearly, it is crucial that workers are sincere when they are making appreciative statements to clients; otherwise there is a danger that the client may experience the interaction as patronising.

Reflective listening
Within the context of MI, reflective listening is a crucial skill and very much more complex than nods or sounds to encourage the client to say more. As noted in relation to open-ended questions, workers try to obtain as much information as possible from the client, and then reflect this back to them in their own words. The reason for this is threefold. It is easier to hear critical things about yourself if spoken in your own words (less likely to sound judgemental), reflecting back on what has just been said may elicit more information, and finally reflecting back may be helpful in clarifying what has been described.

Summarising
This is again a technique that has multiple uses. It can be used to steer the dialogue back if the client is moving away from the subject, or to collect together all of the thoughts the client has expressed about the behaviour, or to sum the situation up, again using the client's own words as far as possible. All of the above, when used together, should elicit talk about change from the client. While the evidence does not support that this is all that is required (Amrehein *et al.* 2003), we do know that change does not happen at all unless people are talking about it.

CASE STUDY 1

Over the past 2 years, the author has trained approximately 200 staff in either 2- or 3-day introductory courses in MI in the United Kingdom. Participants have largely been working in the voluntary sector, in substance misuse services, with a variety of different staff including ex-service users. The training is focused on developing skills, with the 3-day course also concerned with the utilisation of these skills back in the workplace. This emphasis is an attempt to ensure that skills learnt are transferred back to the workplace.

The course supports the following Drug and Alcohol National Occupational Standards units (DANOS) (Federation of Drug and Alcohol Professionals May 2002):

- *AA2 Establish, sustain and disengage from relationships with individuals*
- *AA4 Promote peoples' equality, diversity and rights*
- *AB2 Support individuals who are substance users*
- *AC1 Develop your own knowledge and practice*
- *AC2 Make use of supervision*
- *AC3 Contribute to the development of the knowledge and practice of others*
- *AF2 Carry out assessment to identify and prioritise needs*
- *A11 Counsel individuals about their substance use using recognised theoretical models*

From the beginning, it is acknowledged that many skills are already utilised by staff and that MI places these skills in a certain context with a rationale behind them. Rather than simply hearing a person's story MI is concerned with focusing on the process of change. The training includes a number of methods of teaching. A presentation is followed by a video based on the work of Miller and Rollnick (2002) that displays the skills described in the presentation, and participants then practise those skills in pairs, feeding back on each other's practice.

At the beginning, each participant is asked to think of a change in their behaviour they have been considering. This is the behaviour they will be working with their partner or worker. It is stressed that it is not expected they will change this behaviour, but merely to use it in order to help their partner develop skills as a worker, practising the skills and techniques we will be covering.

In order for participants to work freely and feel safe to divulge information to their partners, it is also stressed that feedback to the whole group does not require that the behaviour is explained to the whole group, but that feedback is concerned with the practice of the techniques. In giving feedback, the participants are asked to give their partners a compliment about their use of the skills, followed by a recommendation and finishing with a further compliment. This structure also enables participants to feel safe in what might, otherwise, be experienced as quite a threatening situation.

While working in pairs, it is important for the trainer to be vigilant about time. Participants are allowed 10 minutes each to work as either 'client' or worker, and are then asked to change roles. Interestingly the usual reluctance experienced by participants when carrying out 'role play' has not, to date, been noted. The opposite has in fact been observed, and it is often difficult to stop people from talking, when working in pairs. This may be a result of the fact that the usual 'acting' component of role play (which some people enjoy, but many dislike intensely) is taken out of the equation. Participants are simply being themselves, either as a person struggling with a behaviour change or as a worker practising skills.

It has been noted with other cohorts of participants, who have been mental health workers, that there appears to be a larger proportion of individuals that have not considered the possibility that behaviour change is difficult. They see clients with mental health problems and associated substance use and believe that ceasing the substance use is a relatively simplistic matter. It is hoped that by introducing into training the struggle of changing relatively simple aspects of their own behaviour, they may reflect differently on their clients' use of substances, and gain a greater understanding of some of the complexity involved in behaviour change.

At the beginning of the training an overview of MI is given, and the opening strategies are introduced. Two tools are then introduced that may help the worker elicit useful information from the client.

The first is the Importance Confidence ruler. This is simply two lines, drawn on a flipchart, with markings of 1–10. The top line is marked Importance and the second Confidence. Participants have already been asked at the beginning to think of a behaviour they would want to change, and without sharing what that behaviour is with the group they are asked to give a number between 1 and 10 of firstly the importance of making that change to them and secondly how confident they are in doing so. They are asked to call out these numbers that are plotted on the flipchart. Invariably the number given to Importance is higher than the number given to Confidence. This may be useful with a client who, for example, gives a score of 8 for Importance, and 2 for Confidence. The client can be asked what would help move them from a 2 to a 3 on the confidence scale. This can be a way of breaking the change process into smaller parts, and forming more realistic goals.

The second tool is to work with the client to draw up a list of what is good and what is not so good about their substance use (pros and cons). It is important to approach this in this particular order as the client is left with the not so good things, which may help to develop discrepancy. This creates what is referred to as cognitive dissonance, which leaves the client feeling uncomfortable and shifts them towards making changes. An advantage of using this tool is that it helps the client to become more realistic about how their substance use is affecting them. This process also facilitates greater insight on the part of the worker as to what issues need to be prioritised.

A video on motivational interviewing (Motivational Interviewing. Professional Training Videotape series) is then shown, demonstrating some of the opening strategies followed by work in pairs on their given behaviours. The feedback process is carefully managed so that the awareness gained can be applied and intergrated into the workers' practice. Then the group examines and explores ways in which these techniques when used together can elicit self-motivational statements. This is followed by a presentation, video, and by an opportunity to practise the additional techniques and to receive further feedback.

Resistance is handled slightly differently. The presentation of techniques to handle resistant behaviour and the video displaying how to use them are still used, but rather than looking at the behaviour they have been working on with their partners, they are asked to think about a situation they have recently experienced where they were resistant. This exercise is either carried out as a whole group or as smaller groups depending on the number of participants. Once again they are not asked to share the situation (although some choose to do so) but to describe and discuss as a group the behaviours that were displayed, what increased their resistance and what helped reduce it.

The formal cycle of MI is then completed with participants formulating a change plan with each other's assistance, following a presentation and video looking at how to proceed. Participants then give feedback to each other in the same format, a compliment on their practice and a recommendation, followed by a further compliment.

If the training has taken place over 3 days, there is time to examine how these skills have been utilised (or not) in the workplace. If the participants have been able to practise, detailed case discussions enable participants to understand and tease out their practice further. If it has not been possible to utilise the skills, it is just as important to discuss this as a group in order to gain ideas as to how to overcome these difficulties. Interestingly, resistance to practicing these skills in the workplace appears to be rare.

Feedback from participants

To date, all feedback on the training has been consistently good. They are asked for three elements that have been identified as being useful about the training and three things which could have been improved.

A comment made in the feedback process was that 'if someone is precontemplative we are not expected to "cure" them and this feels very liberating'. This is significant as so often staff feel that they have failed if a patient does not leave the service drug free.

Conclusion

From the feedback, it seems apparent that mental health staff may well benefit from training in MI in much the same way as drug workers. Of particular interest is the comment, which appeared on a number of occasions, that if someone was precontemplative, staff were not expected to 'cure' them. As mentioned previously, there is sometimes in a mental health setting the expectation that an individual should simply stop substance use. While this may be the most beneficial goal for the patient, it is not necessarily the most realistic. It is at this point when staff may become overwhelmed by the scale of the task that unrealistic goals and expectations are proposed. If the patient then does not manage to achieve them, the quality of the therapeutic relationship may be damaged. Enabling staff to assess where someone is in the cycle of change and reaching mutually acceptable goals are more likely to preserve this relationship. This is not just because the patient is more likely to achieve the goals, which in itself would increase the workers confidence, but also in the event of the goals not being reached, there is more likelihood of future collaboration.

In addition, it is clear that there is scope to investigate the usefulness of this type of training in a systematic way. It would be of particular interest to focus on style of delivery (i.e. if the style of delivery is MI consistent, it is more likely that practice is more influenced on return to the workplace). Many of the comments above would perhaps suggest that the training is delivered in an MI consistent way. Examples of this are the style of the facilitator, the use of summarising and recapping, dealing with resistance, and an increase in confidence in dealing with this way of working.

The use of evidence-based MI interventions in working with dual diagnosis patients is of particular importance. This is because it is an intrinsically empowering way of working that utilises the users' agenda in a non-confrontatative style of working. Importantly, it optimizes the self-esteem of both users and staff.

References

Amrehein PC, Miller WR, Yahne CE, Palmer M, Fulcher L (2003) Client commitment language during motivational interviewing predicts drug use outcomes. *Journal of Consulting and Clinical Psychology* 71(5): 862–878.

Drug and Alcohol National Occupational Standards (DANOS) (2002) *Federation of Drug and Alcohol Professionals*. London: Drugscope.

Miller W, Rollnick S (2002) *Motivational Interviewing: Preparing People for Change*, 2nd Edition. New York, London: The Guildford Press.

Motivational Interviewing. Professional Training Videotape Series. *Tape A. Introduction to Motivational Interviewing*.

Noonan WC, Moyers TB (1997) Motivational Interviewing: A review. *Journal of Substance Misuse* 2: 8–16.

Prochaska JO, DiClemente CC (1984) *The Transtheoretical Approach: Crossing the Traditional Boundaries of Therapy*. Malabar, FL: Kreiger.

Project MATCH Research Group (1997) Matching alcoholism treatments to client heterogeneity: Project MATCH posttreatment drinking outcomes. *Journal of Studies on Alcohol* 58: 7–29.

Resnicow K, Dilorio C, Soet J, Borrelli B, Ernst D, Hecht J (2001) Motivational interviewing in health promotion. It sounds like something is changing. *Health Psychology*, 21: 444–451.

Chapter 7

Psychological Interventions

Patrick Callaghan and David Jones

Introduction

People living with a dual diagnosis often have complex needs. Consequently, it is unlikely that a single intervention will have much impact on meeting their needs. Although the focus of this chapter is psychological interventions, there is a move towards recommending an integrated approach to the care and treatment of people living with a dual diagnosis, delivered as part of mainstream mental health services (Department of Health 2002, 2006; Hussein Rassool 2002; Ziedonis *et al.* 2005). This approach derives largely from assertive-community treatment (ACT) models such as those developed in New Hampshire (Drake *et al.* 1998) and New York (Hellerstein *et al.* 1995). These approaches include not only psychological interventions but also pharmacological, social and motivational interventions. In this chapter, we will outline the nature of psychological interventions, examine the evidence for their use and demonstrate how mental health professionals can use these interventions in practice.

The nature and type of psychological interventions

Psychology is the study of mental processes and behaviour. Mental processes include cognition, memory, intelligence, personality, perception, sensation, beliefs, attitudes, information processing, thoughts and speech. The aim of psychological interventions is to effect a change in the way people interpret their experiences, thus enabling a corresponding change in their behaviour and aiding in their recovery from incapacitating mental health problems. For example, we recognise the importance of cognitive functioning to changing behaviour, and of maintaining this change. People affected by severe mental health problems such as dual diagnosis often report deficits in cognitive functioning. Impairments to memory, attention, and thought processes will impair a person's ability to use recommended cognitive and behavioural skills necessary to change how they cope with distressing symptoms, and associated substance use. Psychological interventions may be cognitive and behavioural, psychodynamic or humanistic, including variations of these, centred on working individually, or in groups, with individuals, their families and significant others. Sometimes, the terms psychotherapy and counselling are used to describe psychological interventions. As Chapter 6 of this book deals with motivational interviewing, we have excluded this 'intervention' from our consideration here.

The evidence for psychological interventions in dual diagnosis

There is a sound evidence base demonstrating the effectiveness of many forms of psychological interventions for many types of mental health problems (see Lambert 2003; Roth & Fonagy 2004, for example). However, the evidence underpinning the use of psychological interventions for dual diagnosis varies, and this is largely due to the move towards integrated services in which psychological interventions are offered as part of these services and are seldom evaluated independently of the integrated approach. Studies investigating the impact of psychological interventions either as part of an integrated approach or as a specific intervention to address a specific outcome demonstrate the promise of such interventions to enable clients to attain and maintain abstinence from using substances (Drake & Mueser 2000), reduce health care costs (Jerrell & Ridgely 1997) and minimise the impact of symptoms on activities of living (Meuser *et al.* 2003). Following their systematic review of studies of psychosocial treatment programmes for the Cochrane Collaboration, Jeffery *et al.* (2000) conclude that there is no reliable evidence supporting the use of these programmes in treating people with dual diagnosis. A persuasive case is made for the use of cognitive behavioural integrated treatment (C-BIT) (Graham 2004), but the evidence behind this approach is unclear. In *Integrated Treatment for Dual Disorders: A Manual for Clinicians Working with Clients Diagnosed with Mental Health and Substance Use Problems*, Mueser and colleagues demonstrate the successful application of interventions such as cognitive behavioural counselling, stage-wise case management and motivational interviewing (Mueser *et al.* 2003).

In the absence of a strong evidence base underpinning psychological interventions in the care and treatment of dual diagnosis, good practice guidelines have been formulated in the United States and the United Kingdom. These guidelines were derived from the consensus views of experts working in the field (Department of Health 2002, 2006; Ziedonis *et al.* 2005).

In the next part of this chapter, we describe the use of psychological interventions in promoting recovery in people with dual diagnosis.

Abou-Saleh (2004) suggests that a common tendency is to treat the co-morbid disorder as secondary to the primary disorder and to assume that the secondary disorder will improve as a result of treatment of the first. This might explain why the emphasis in the dual diagnosis literature is on the effectiveness of substance use interventions and less on 'psychiatric' interventions. Indeed, in an excellent review of controlled trials in this field, Drake *et al.* (2007) state that almost all the studies that they reviewed are based on the addition of a substance use intervention to a normal mental health programme, adding that, 'because the intervention for substance use disorder defines the experimental manipulation in these studies, substance use or some consequence of substance use logically becomes the primary outcome.' Even though many studies also examine other outcome domains, this still suggests that the focus in dual diagnosis research remains on substance use as the primary problem with secondary psychiatric consequences, which would appear to ignore the three other subtypes of dual diagnosis identified by Lehman *et al.* (1989). In turn, this would appear to steer researchers away from evaluating mainstream interventions for mental health problems of people with dual diagnosis.

The American Psychological Association Presidential Task Force on Evidence-Based Practice (2006) defined an evidence-based treatment as one that has been shown to be effective in at least two randomised controlled trials that are of sound methodology. If we accept this definition, many interventions would be excluded from the dual diagnosis evidence base owing to the methodological problems identified by Jeffery *et al.* (2000) – many studies that would appear to be examining the same problem use different methodologies or outcomes. This leads to the classic dilemma for clinicians – what to do in the absence of evidence-based treatments? Do we integrate into our practice interventions that have been researched for 'single' diagnoses? This, in itself, can prove problematic. The two largest studies of effective psychological interventions in the alcohol field do not prove particularly helpful to the dual diagnosis clinician. Project MATCH (Project MATCH Research Group, 1993) and the United Kingdom Alcohol Treatment Trial (UKATT Research Team, 2001) both specifically excluded people who had serious mental health problems.

Another issue that affects the clinician is how effective interventions translate from research into clinical practice. While highlighting the strengths of the research of Barrowclough *et al.* (2001), James *et al.* (2004) point out the practical difficulties faced when trying to integrate such a broad-reaching package of interventions into routine practice, and also mention the cost in terms of resources.

A further issue to be considered is, what do we want the psychological intervention to achieve? Do we want it to be the treatment in itself or enhance the effectiveness of other psychological interventions? Motivational approaches have been used to enhance compliance with medication regimes (Kemp *et al.* 1996) and with attending out-patient treatment itself (Swanson *et al.* 1999). Motivational interviewing is discussed in more detail in Chapter 6. Indeed, some of the strongest treatment effects come from packages that incorporate a number of psychological interventions (see Barrowclough *et al.* 2001; Bellack *et al.* 2006). This is likely to be a very important point for clinicians, since it can be expected that substance users presenting in psychiatric services who have not actually requested help for their substance misuse will be much more suitable for motivational intervention in the first instance rather than other therapies that assume that a person is already ready to change.

Individual therapies

Drake *et al.* (2007) suggest that most of the randomised controlled trials that have been conducted on individual therapies for dual diagnosis have been based on motivational interviewing or have at least included motivational interviewing as a core component, e.g. Barrowclough *et al.* (2001), and that the evidence to support their effectiveness is 'relatively weak or inconsistent'.

A lack of evaluation of progress on psychiatric symptoms is a common feature among many studies in this field, with the exceptions of Barrowclough *et al.* (2001) and Baker *et al.* (2006). Baker *et al.* (2006) combined motivational interviewing with cognitive behaviour therapy and relapse prevention. Barrowclough *et al.* (2001) also added family interventions. Both studies showed not only a short-term reduction in substance use but also a gradual reversion over 12–18 months to previous levels of use. However, both studies also showed improvements in general functioning and depression over 12–18 months. This suggests that repeated use of these interventions is required over time. Once again, it is not possible to separate out the effects of different types of intervention, or even if there were other factors at play, such as increased contact time with a clinician for the intervention group.

Group therapies

Mueser and Drake (2005) state that there have been a number of evaluations of group treatment that have proven more effective than no intervention or standard 12-step approaches. Drake *et al.* (2007) conclude from their systematic review that group counselling interventions produce strong results in terms of reducing substance use and improving other domains, but that they appear to be of limited effectiveness when it comes to non-substance use psychopathology. Given that most studies treat substance use as the main experimental variable, perhaps this outcome is unsurprising.

Most group therapy programmes appear to incorporate a variety of approaches. For example, Bellack *et al.* (2006) combined cognitive behaviour therapy, skills training and contingency management to produce significantly better results than a standard treatment in terms of less frequent drug use, survival in treatment, attendance at treatment sessions, reduced hospital admissions and quality of life.

While group therapy research interventions appear to produce stronger outcomes than individual interventions, a common feature of group therapy research is a very high attrition rate, with even studies that show good success still losing a third of subjects (Bellack *et al.* 2006), which would still be of concern to clinicians.

One study that did appear to tackle the issue of high drop-out rates (James *et al.* 2004) was conducted within the context of a case management system (which once again makes it difficult to separate the effectiveness of the intervention from the framework) and also used payment for attendance at follow-up appointments, which is likely to have implications for most clinical services. This study was also one of the few to assess the impact of the intervention on mental health symptoms of subjects.

Cognitive behaviour therapy and relapse prevention

Cognitive behaviour therapy is a well-established and evidence-based approach to the treatment of both mental health (Grant *et al.* 2004) and substance use problems (Conrod & Stewart 2005).

Relapse prevention refers to a cognitive behavioural approach to promote the maintenance of desired goals and behaviours. The model is well supported in the substance use field as an evidence-based treatment (see McGovern & Carroll 2003). However, there have been virtually no evaluations of the approach for people with a dual diagnosis. McGovern and Carroll (2003) state that most of the dual diagnosis treatment research has focused on engagement and building motivation to change rather than the maintenance stage of change.

Given the inter-related nature of the problems experienced by people who have a dual diagnosis and the emphasis on integrated treatment, it seems helpful to heed the advice of McGovern *et al.* (2005) when they suggest that, 'Relapse prevention therapy can be more broadly conceptualised and focused on lifestyle change and recovery rather than simple substance use or abstinence'.

While there are no well-validated randomised controlled studies in this area, a number of smaller-scale studies and treatment manuals do show promise.

Schmitz *et al.* (2002) showed cognitive behavioural therapy (CBT) plus medication management to be superior to medication management in bipolar patients who also had a substance use disorder when it came to mood symptom reduction and compliance with medication, although it made no difference to substance use.

The C-BIT Treatment Manual (Graham 2004) provides a useful integration and application to dual diagnosis of evidence-based interventions from the broader substance use and cognitive behaviour therapy fields, and has been used by other researchers when devising their own intervention programmes, e.g. Baker *et al.* (2006).

Family interventions

Family interventions aim to raise the knowledge, supportiveness and coping skills of the family members. To date, only Barrowclough *et al.* (2001) have evaluated family interventions for dual diagnosis in the context of a randomised controlled trial, and this took place in the context of a broad-reaching package of care. Again, the clinician is left to draw upon studies from both fields and try to integrate the best of both.

Contingency management

Contingency management is a treatment that aims to modify target behaviours (in this case substance use) by the systematic provision or withholding of rewards. In the substance use and dual diagnosis fields, contingency management usually refers to rewards for maintaining abstinence from substance use, normally assessed by urinalysis, e.g. Drebing *et al.* (2005); Bellack *et al.* (2006). It has been found to increase the duration of abstinence. This approach appears to show some promise, although when it has been suggested for routine clinical use in the United Kingdom, it has proven controversial (BBC 2007). Bellack *et al.* (2006), however, do argue for the usefulness of urinalysis contingency, suggesting that the average cost ranged from US$7–10 for the urinalysis plus the financial reinforcement. In non-dual diagnosis populations, it has shown benefits with problem cocaine users in terms of retention in treatment and social outcomes such as employment and reduced drug and alcohol use (Higgins *et al.* 2003).

Conclusion

There is clearly a great need for more high-quality research in the dual diagnosis field, especially when it comes to establishing which psychological interventions are effective, both within and without the context of integrated treatment services of varying international flavours.

Whether it is a function of the uncertainty created by a lack of robust evidence for this client group or an organisational unwillingness to fund appropriate training or simply a parsimonious approach to treatment, it might well be the case that 'at the practice level, effective psychosocial interventions are rarely used and ineffective pharmacological interventions are overused' (Mueser & Drake 2007).

Haddock *et al.* (2003), in reporting the 18-month outcomes from the same study as Barrowclough *et al.* (2001), reported that after 18 months, subjects in the intervention group had superior general functioning and negative symptom scores, and that there was no difference from the control group on percentage of days of abstinence from illicit drugs and alcohol. Schmitz *et al.* (2002) found similarly that substance use remained largely unaffected by their intervention, although other areas of functioning improved.

This seems to reinforce the point made earlier in this chapter that substance use outcomes should not necessarily be the main focus of research, and possibly represents the oversimplification of an answer to a complex problem.

References

Abou-Saleh MT (2004) Dual diagnosis: management within a psychosocial context. *Advances in Psychiatric Treatment* 10: 352–360.

American Psychological Association Presidential Task Force on Evidence-Based Practice. (2006) Evidence-based practice in psychology. *American Psychologist* 61: 271–285.

Baker A, Bucci S, Lewin TJ, *et al.* (2006) Cognitive–behavioural therapy for substance use disorders in people with psychotic disorders: Randomised controlled trial. *British Journal of Psychiatry* 188: 439–448.

Barrowclough C, Haddock G, Tarrier N, *et al.* (2001) Randomized controlled trial of motivational interviewing, cognitive behavior therapy, and family intervention for patients with comorbid schizophrenia and substance use disorders. *American Journal of Psychiatry* 158: 1706–1713.

BBC (2007) Shopping voucher plan for addicts. Available at http://news.bbc.co.uk/1/hi/health/6294795.stm Last updated on 26.01.07. (Accessed on 19.12.07)

Bellack AS, Bennett ME, Gearon JS, *et al.* (2006) A randomized clinical trial of a new behavioral treatment of drug abuse in people with severe and persistent mental illness. *Archives of General Psychiatry* 63: 426–432.

Conrod PJ, Stewart SH (2005) A critical look at dual-focused cognitive-behavioral treatments for comorbid substance use and psychiatric disorders: strengths, limitations, and future directions. *Journal of Cognitive Psychotherapy* 19 (3): 261–284.

Department of Health (2002) *Mental Health Policy Implementation Guide: Dual Diagnosis: Good Practice.* London: Department of Health.

Department of Health (2006) *Dual Diagnosis in Mental Health Inpatient and Day Hospital Settings: Guidance on the Assessment and Management of Patients in*

Mental Health Inpatient and Day Hospital Settings Who Have Mental Ill-Health and Substance Use Problems. London: Department of Health.

Drake RE, McHugo GJ, Clark RE, *et al.* (1998) Assertive community treatment for patients with co-occurring severe mental illness and substance use disorder: a clinical trial. *American Journal of Orthopsychiatry* 68 (2): 201–215.

Drake RE, Mueser KT (2000) Psychosocial approaches to dual diagnosis. *Schizophrenia Bulletin* 26 (1): 105.

Drake RE, O'Neal EL, Wallach MA (2007) A systematic review of psychosocial research on psychosocial interventions for people with co-occurring severe mental and substance use disorders. *Journal of Substance Abuse Treatment* 34: 123–138.

Drebing CE, Van Ormer EA, Krebs C, *et al.* (2005) The impact of enhanced incentives on vocational rehabilitation outcomes for dually diagnosed veterans. *Journal of Applied Behavioral Analysis* 38: 359–372.

Graham HL (2004) *Cognitive-Behavioural Integrated Treatment (C-BIT): A Treatment Manual for Substance Misuse in People with Severe Mental Health Problems*. Chichester, UK: John Wiley and Sons.

Grant A, Mills J, Mulhern RP, Short N (eds) (2004) *Cognitive Behavioural Therapy in Mental Health Care*. London: Sage.

Haddock G, Barrowclough C, Tarrier N *et al.* (2003) Cognitive behavioural therapy and motivational intervention for schizophrenia and substance misuse: 18-month outcomes of a randomised controlled trial. *British Journal of Psychiatry* 183: 418–426.

Hellerstein DJ, Rosenthal RN, Miner CR (1995) A prospective study of integrated outpatient treatment for substance abusing schizophrenic patients. *American Journal on Addictions* 4 (1): 33–42.

Higgins ST, Sigmon SC, Wong CJ, *et al.* (2003) Community reinforcement therapy for cocaine-dependent outpatients. *Archives of General Psychiatry* 60: 1043–1052.

Hussein Rassool G (2002) *Dual Diagnosis: Substance Misuse and Psychiatric Disorders*. Oxford: Blackwell Science.

James W, Preston NJ, Koh G, Spencer C, Kisely SR, Castle DJ (2004) A group intervention which assists patients with dual diagnosis reduce their drug use: a randomized controlled trial. *Psychological Medicine* 34 (6): 983–990.

Jeffery DP, Ley A, McLaren S, Siegfried N (2000) Psychosocial programmes for people with both severe mental illness and substance misuse. *Cochrane Database of Systematic Reviews* (2): Art. No. CD001088. DOI:10.1002/14651858.

Jerrell JM, Ridgely MS (1997) Dual diagnosis care for severe and persistent disorders: a comparison of three methods. *Behavioral Healthcare Tomorrow* 6 (3): 26–33.

Kemp R, Hayward P, Applewhaite G, *et al.* (1996) Compliance therapy in psychotic patients: randomised controlled trial. *BMJ* 312: 345–349.

Lambert MJ (2003) *Bergin and Garfield's Handbook of Psychotherapy and Behavior Change*, 5th Edition. London: John Wiley and Sons.

Lehman AF, Myers CP, Corty E (1989) Assessment and classification of patients with psychiatric and substance abuse syndromes. *Hospital and Community Psychiatry* 131: 1121–1123.

McGovern MP, Carroll KM (2003) Evidence-based practices for substance use disorders. *Psychiatric Clinics of North America* 26: 991–1010.

McGovern MP, Wrisley BR, Drake RE (2005) Relapse of substance use disorder and its prevention among persons with co-occurring disorders. *Psychiatric Services* 56: 1270–1273.

Mueser KT, Drake RE (2005) Psychosocial interventions for adults with severe mental illnesses and co-occurring substance use disorders: a review of specific interventions. *Journal of Dual Diagnosis* 1 (2): 57–82.

Mueser KT, Drake RE (2007) Comorbidity: what have we learned and where are we going? *Clinical Psychology: Science and Practice* 14 (1): 64–69.

Mueser KT, Noordsy DL, Drake RE, Fox L (2003) *Integrated Treatment for Dual Disorders: A Manual for Clinicians Working with Clients Diagnosed with Mental Health and Substance Use Problems*. New York: Guildford Press.

Mueser KT, Torrey WC, Lynde D, Singer P, Drake RE (2003) Implementing evidence-based practices for people with severe mental illness. *Behavior Modification* 27: 387–411.

Project MATCH Research Group (1993) Project MATCH: rationale and methods for a multisite clinical trial matching alcoholism patients to treatment. *Alcoholism: Clinical and Experimental Research* 17: 1130–1145.

Roth A, Fonagy P (2004) *What Works for Whom? A Critical Review of Psychotherapy Research*, 2nd Edition. London: Guildford Publications.

Schmitz JM, Averill P, Sayre S, *et al.* (2002) Cognitive–behavioral treatment of bipolar disorder and substance abuse: a preliminary randomized study. *Addiction Disorders & Their Treatment* 1: 17–24.

Swanson AJ, Pantalon MV, Cohen KR, *et al.* (1999) Motivational interviewing and treatment adherence among psychiatric and dually diagnosed patients. *Journal of Nervous & Mental Disease* 187: 630–635.

UKATT Research Team (2001) United Kingdom alcohol treatment trial (UKATT): hypotheses, design and methods. *Alcohol and Alcoholism* 36 (1): 11–21.

Ziedonis DM, Smelson D, Rosenthal RN, *et al.* (2005) Improving the care of individuals with schizophrenia and substance use disorders: consensus recommendations. *Journal of Psychiatric Practice* 11 (5): 315–339.

Chapter 8

Alcohol and Mood Disorders

Julie Attenborough

Introduction

In discussions and investigation of dual diagnosis, the association between alcohol and mood disorder is found to be particularly strong. In keeping with the almost universal use of alcohol in Western society, the prevalence of alcohol problems far exceeds the problems associated with other drugs. In the United Kingdom alcohol consumption is rising, doubling between 1960 and 2002, while the price of alcohol relative to income has fallen by a half (PMSU 2004). There is evidence that all of the psychiatric disorders are more likely to occur in people with alcohol problems than those without (Helzer & Pryzbeck 1988). The prevalence of mood disorder in hospitalised alcoholics has been found to be between 8 and 53% (Roy 1996).

In clinical practice there is difficulty in distinguishing between alcohol-induced mood disorders, depression secondary to alcohol withdrawal, independent depressive episodes and the use of alcohol for self-medication that is seen with both depressed and elated mood. In 2002, the Department of Health (DH 2002) issued guidance on how services should be delivered for people who have both mental illness and alcohol problems, directing that mental health services will have primary responsibility for individuals with severe and enduring mental illness (mainstreaming).

Harm, alcohol and mental illness

There is a considerable raised risk of completed suicide in people who have a diagnosis of depression and alcohol dependency (Beck *et al.* 1989). In a study investigating the disproportionate suicidality in patients with major depression and alcoholism, Cornelius *et al.* (1995) compared the clinical profile of patients with a dual diagnosis of alcoholism and depression with that of alcoholics who were not depressed, and depressed patients who were not alcoholic. Patients with dual diagnosis differed only on two specific depressive symptoms – suicidality, which was 59% higher, and low self-esteem, which was 22% higher (Cornelius *et al.* 1995). Indeed, the rate of completed suicides has been demonstrated to be directly related to the per capita consumption of alcohol in the former USSR. A sharp decline in the suicide rate (34.5%) was noted between 1984 and 1988 throughout the USSR. This occurred shortly after strict restrictions were imposed on the sale of alcohol. A regression analysis demonstrated that suicide and alcohol consumption were positively correlated, use of alcohol being implicated in more than 50% of suicides over the whole country (Wasserman *et al.* 1994).

In addition to the experience of having two related diagnoses, people who are diagnosed with mood disorder and alcoholism are more likely to experience homelessness, unemployment and difficulties in maintaining relationships (Hussein Rassool 2006). Compounding this is the constellation of physical and other problems prevalent in people who use large amounts of alcohol over a prolonged period.

Owing to associated disinhibition, people who use alcohol are also at increased risk of self-harm, and this is compounded by low mood in depression, as uncomfortable thoughts and feelings are unleashed. Therefore, self-harm as opposed to attempted suicide generally occurs when the person is intoxicated. Madden (1994) has suggested that long-term alcohol ingestion also promotes a sustained phase of depression, both as a coping mechanism to deal with problems and difficulties and through physiological changes.

Presentation: alcohol and mental illness

There is evidence that prolonged use of large amounts of alcohol may exacerbate some of the symptoms of depression. Sleep pattern and quality are affected by alcohol use, although intoxication with alcohol may assist with the initial insomnia sometimes experienced in depression, the patient falling asleep in a drunken stupor. Early morning wakening is likely to be experienced by people who use large amounts of alcohol, whether depressed or not. Mood may be altered, and when diurnal variation in mood is present, the low mood in the morning may be exacerbated by withdrawal symptoms, and an increased need for relief drinking, a maintenance factor in alcohol dependence. Alcohol ingestion may worsen difficulties with concentration experienced as part of an affective illness due to cognitive impairment.

Alcohol use can affect appetite. Many chronic alcohol users experience gastritis and may substitute alcohol for food. Nutrients are less well absorbed and the additional complication of appetite disturbance in mood disorder, particularly depression, means that patients with dual diagnosis are at increased risk of developing nutritional deficiencies, which can lead to Wernicke–Korsakoff syndrome and anaemia.

Loss of libido is common in depressive episodes, and alcohol abuse can itself cause high rates of sexual dysfunction (Bhui & Puffett 1994). Alcohol use is also implicated in relationship problems, compounding the sexual dysfunction experienced. Seventy-five percent of subjects in one sample had premature ejaculation, delayed ejaculation, low libido and persistent erectile dysfunction (Schover 1988). These findings are partly due to the physiological sequelae of prolonged alcohol use, such as peripheral neuropathy and cognitive impairment, and partly due to the direct sedative effect of alcohol on the central nervous system. These effects are unlikely to improve even after a prolonged period of abstinence.

It is also important to note that the disinhibiting effects of alcohol not only increase the possibility of impulsive acts, such as self-harming behaviour, but also increase the risk of sexual risk-taking. The use of condoms has been shown to be reduced in people who are intoxicated with alcohol. There is an increased likelihood of multiple partners (Ericksen & Trocki 1994). This is an issue for people who are depressed, but particularly significant for people who are hypomanic and may be sexually disinhibited with impaired judgement.

Alcohol use in bipolar and unipolar disorders is associated with a poor prognosis. This has been demonstrated even when the mood disorder predates the alcohol problem (O'Connel *et al.* 1991). People experiencing hypomania or mania may use alcohol as a sedative in order to sleep or relax, and may lack judgement about the quantity of alcohol to ingest. Use of alcohol as self-medication for symptom relief is also a factor in depressed people, although some may reduce their intake because of impaired social functioning and anhedonia. In an article examining the effects of alcohol on social responses and self-awareness, Steele *et al.* (1990) discuss the effect of alcohol on perception and thought, distinguishing between the direct pharmaceutical effects of alcohol and what is described as an alcohol myopia, in relation to social responses and self-perception. The patient develops a distorted view of their own social functioning and has pseudo-insights into their situation, which are not accurate.

Medication and dual diagnosis

Those people who are treated for depressive illness and who continue to drink can experience further problems. Some antidepressants potentiate the effects of alcohol, so that the patient experiences intoxication and loss of control at an earlier stage. It has been demonstrated that the effectiveness of some antidepressants is impaired by continued alcohol use (Ciraulo & Barnhill 1988). Psychotropic medication and continued alcohol use may also exacerbate gastritis and liver disease related to alcohol use. Depressed patients who are suicidal or at risk of self-harm may overdose

on antidepressants or lithium. Although the introduction of selective serotonin reuptake inhibitors (SSRIs) has reduced the risk of fatal overdose
considerably, older tricyclic antidepressants are still prescribed.

The symptoms of anxiety and depression are common among people
entering alcohol treatment programmes (Raistrick *et al.* 2006). Evidence considered in the review of the effectiveness of treatment for alcohol problems
(Raistrick *et al.* 2006) suggests that up to 80% of problem drinkers going into
treatment have clinically significant symptoms.

Alcohol use in patients with dual diagnosis is often considered to be
internally controlled, and so disulfiram (Antabuse) is not often prescribed.
Borup and Unden (1994) assessed the outcome of treating patients with
dual diagnosis with a combination of an antidepressant (fluoxetine) and
disulfiram, with good results. Seventy percent of the depressed patients
improved considerably. However, there is no convincing evidence that the
use of antidepressants can treat alcohol dependence (Torrens *et al.* 2005;
Raistrick *et al.* 2006). It is important to note that disulfiram is contraindicated
in people with a history of psychosis, cerebrovascular accident and any
cardiovascular problems because of its potential to induce hypertensive crisis.
For the same reason, it is also contraindicated in pregnancy (Parker *et al.* 2008).

It has also been suggested (Lamb 1982) that people who have a psychiatric
diagnosis such as unipolar or bipolar affective disorder and use substances
problematically may be seeking an identity that is more acceptable and less
stigmatising than that of a psychiatric patient, and that having a substance
problem is more normal and mainstream than being considered mad by
society.

There is general agreement in the literature that excessive use of alcohol
generally precedes mood disorder (Schuckit 1986; Bakken *et al.* 2003). In a
large study of 2945 alcohol-dependant people, Schuckit *et al.* (1997) found it
possible to distinguish between alcohol-induced and independent depressive
episodes in people dependent on alcohol, discovering that those who had
independent episodes were more likely to be female, married, Caucasian, to
have had less treatment for their alcohol problem and to have a close relative
with a major mood disorder. This finding has important implications for
treatment of people with alcohol problems and mood disorder.

The symptoms of depression are often present during, and shortly
after, withdrawal from alcohol, although these will generally remit within
1–2 weeks of abstinence. Raistrick (2000) suggests that up to 80% of problem drinkers entering into treatment present with mental health symptoms
that are not present after a period of abstinence. Chemical treatment for
depressive illness is not indicated at this time, although it has been suggested
(Rubinstein *et al.* 1990) that secondary depression induced by alcohol is often
mistakenly treated with antidepressants. However, identifying a depressive
illness in people being treated for alcoholism is problematic, as symptoms of

withdrawal can mimic depressive symptoms. Schuckit and Maristela (1988) discusses the difficulties in distinguishing between drinking and alcoholism, sadness and depression and anxious feelings and anxiety disorders. He suggests that the primary disorder should be arrived at by an analysis of the chronology of the symptoms experienced by the patient. Gorman (1992) suggests that primary and secondary alcoholism should be distinguished using behavioural criteria such as giving up of interests and activities to spend time drinking, rather than by the presence of alcohol-related problems and withdrawal phenomena.

Green (1996) describes her personal experience of treatment for bipolar affective disorder and alcohol and drug problems. Her account clearly demonstrates the difficulty in accessing appropriate help for her problems. Health services are focused on one problem or another, even when they are so closely interrelated. Her account also describes her experience of an integrated dual diagnosis programme that successfully treated her problems, incorporating a holistic model of care.

CASE STUDY 1

Sidney, a white English man, was born in Liverpool in 1940 and was the son of a dockworker and cleaner. He experienced a difficult childhood; he was first born, conceived shortly before his father went away to fight in the war. In 1944, after his father returned, a second child, Peter was born. Sidney felt that his father favoured Peter, and the combination of Peter's arrival and his father's return to the family home meant that Sidney could no longer share the bed with his mother. His father was a disciplinarian and a heavy drinker, and Sidney's childhood was characterised by arguments and violent beatings. Holmes and Robins (1987) examined the influence of disciplinary experience in childhood on the development of alcohol problems and depression in later life. They studied 200 people between 18 and 49 years from a population with a diagnosis of depression and alcoholism. Unfair, inconsistent and harsh discipline in childhood were identified as predictors of alcohol and depressive disorders, independent of the influence of genetics, sex and childhood behaviour problems.

Sidney passed his 11+ and progressed to Grammar School, but was a poor achiever, and when the relationship with his father deteriorated he began to despair and had thoughts of suicide. He continued to experience severe beatings from his father, which in adolescence was further associated with depressive symptoms, alcohol abuse and suicidal ideation in later life (as discussed by Straus & Kantor 1994). His self-esteem was very low and at the age of 14 he began to drink his father's whisky in the evenings when his father was out at the pub. The effect of the intoxication with whisky was to relieve the anxiety that Sidney felt about his father's return from the pub, and it helped him feel more confident. When his father discovered that Sidney had been drinking, a violent argument ensued, resulting in Sidney leaving home at the age of 15 and joining the merchant navy. Here he was exposed to a drinking culture and began to drink very heavily and experience periods of depression. However, he felt happier than he had done at home and decided to join the Royal Navy at 18. He trained to be a mechanic in the Navy and for 8 years experienced stability.

Sidney left the Royal Navy at the age of 26 and returned to Liverpool. He met Jane, whom he married after 6 months. He became a long-distance lorry driver and spent long periods away from home. He found the return to civilian life very stressful and had little contact with his family. Jane and Sidney had two children, a boy and a girl. Sidney started to drink heavily shortly after the birth of his second child. He drank alone at home, rather than in the pub. He experienced withdrawal symptoms early in the morning and would have a drink to 'steady himself' before driving for the day.

After a heavy drinking bout Sidney had to drive to London to deliver some bricks. He drank half a bottle of whisky before setting out, but did not feel intoxicated. On the motorway he was involved in a road traffic accident in which a woman and her baby were killed. He was not breathalysed at the scene of the accident, nor did the police blame him for causing the accident. However, because he knew he had ingested so much alcohol, Sidney felt he was responsible.

Subsequently, Sidney's drinking increased. His relationship with Jane deteriorated, he was unable to sustain an erection and began to develop a depressive illness. He took a large overdose of barbiturates and alcohol in his lorry one night, leaving a note for Jane apologising for abandoning her with so much responsibility, but saying that he could not live with what he had done and could see no future. He was discovered by a policeman, taken to hospital and survived. He was assessed by a psychiatrist, considered to be clinically depressed and at risk of killing himself and admitted to hospital informally. He remained in hospital for 2 years.

In investigating the aetiology of secondary depression in alcoholics, Roy (1996) considered the role of life events. Brown and Harris (1978) demonstrated that women are more likely to develop a depressive illness if they had experienced a life event or chronic adversity. Roy studied 40 depressed men with alcoholism as the primary diagnosis and compared them with matched controls who had a primary diagnosis of depression. He found that in the 6 months before developing the depression, alcoholics had experienced more life events than the control group, more negative life events, and significantly, more events caused by alcohol. They were also more likely to have attempted suicide.

It is likely that Sidney's experience in the accident contributed to this depressive episode. While in hospital, Sidney was abstinent from alcohol, and investigations found that he had signs of liver disease. This was reversible, and the period of abstinence improved his physical and mental state. He was discharged and went home to live with Jane and the children. The relationship quickly broke down, and 18 months later Sidney left Jane and travelled to London seeking work. He never saw her or the children again. He was 36.

Sidney enrolled with a care agency that found him work in a residential care home for people with severe mental and physical disabilities. He enjoyed the work, but once again found himself in a heavy drinking environment. He had sex with three of his female colleagues within 2 months of starting the job. He found that he had increased amounts of energy, could work for 12-hour days and then go out drinking without experiencing any problems. He began to feel very confident with an inflated view of his own self-importance. He began to make plans to open his own chain of residential care homes and drew up complicated plans of how they would work, including diagrams. He talked to whoever would listen to him about his ideas. Colleagues noticed that he was talking very rapidly, and much of what he said did not make sense. He found it more and more difficult to sleep and was often pacing around for most of the night. He drank more alcohol to help him sleep.

After 2 weeks he had noticeably lost weight and often smelled strongly of alcohol. His self-care was very poor, and he appeared to have little awareness of how he presented himself. He propositioned female colleagues, and was quite insistent, boasting of his sexual prowess. One night he was found sitting outside a colleague's room masturbating. He was suspended from duty and told to visit his GP. His GP referred him to a psychiatrist, who diagnosed hypomania. Because of his history of depression Sidney was considered to have bipolar affective disorder.

In hospital he recovered quickly with neuroleptic medication. He found it difficult to resist the urge to drink, especially at night to help him sleep, and he therefore continued to drink half a bottle of spirits every night.

Although there is a paucity of data concerning the effects of alcohol on the efficacy and action of neuroleptics, Bradwejn et al. (1983) have found that when people are drinking heavily, thioridazine leaves the blood quickly, thereby decreasing the amount of tranquilliser in the blood. If the thioridazine is taken with reduced amounts of alcohol, two units being optimal, the levels of thioridazine are increased, thus aiding tranquillisation of the patient. This area clearly needs further investigation as it may add to our understanding of the aetiology of alcohol dependence in people prescribed neuroleptic medication for schizophrenia, although there is far more caution about prescribing thioridazine in recent years.

Sidney stayed in hospital for 8 months and was discharged taking lithium carbonate. He had an outpatient appointment and planned to return to work. When he returned home he found a letter informing him that he had been dismissed from his job because he had not disclosed his history of alcohol dependence and depressive illness. With his job he lost his accommodation and had to go to a direct access resettlement unit in central London. He was allocated a bed in a dormitory inhabited by street drinkers and people with schizophrenia who had predominately negative symptoms. He took his medication for 2 days and then it was stolen from him. He did not have access to health care; a visiting medical officer (VMO) attended the resettlement unit once a week, but there was always a very long wait to see him, and Sidney had been told that the VMO was not sympathetic to people with mental health problems. He tried to find work, but whenever he gave his address as the resettlement unit he was turned down. Welfare agencies set up to help ex-servicemen said that they could not help homeless people when he approached them.

Sidney began to feel very angry about his situation. He could not accept that he had a serious mental illness or that he had an alcohol problem. He was very resistant to approaching any agencies for help, and few existed that offered a service to people with complex needs who were homeless. He surveyed the other men in the hostel and felt that he could end his days there, drinking heavily, and becoming like the men he saw with schizophrenia who lay on their beds all day, muttering to themselves. He did not understand the nature of his illness or the implications of his diagnosis.

Epidemiological studies of the prevalence of mental health and substance problems in homeless people in Britain have focused on hostel dwelling men, as they are more accessible than the street homeless population. Timms and Fry (1989) found that 30% of men in a hostel had schizophrenia, 8% had alcoholism, 3% affective disorder and 7% personality disorder. Power and Attenborough (2003) reported that homeless people with mental health problems who were also dependent on alcohol were five times more likely to lose contact with services than those who did not have a concurrent alcohol problem. The effect of living in a chaotic environment inhabited by people with untreated mental health problems must be assumed to be detrimental to recovery from a recent depressive episode, complicated by alcohol dependence.

Sidney felt utterly alone and began to ruminate about the past – the guilt he felt about the accident, leaving Jane and his relationship with his father, who had always said that he was a worthless individual. Sidney stopped eating; he could not face the food in the hostel. He woke up early in the morning, dreading the day ahead; he could see no future. He began to spend his days in the parks of London drinking whatever he could afford to buy or beg for. One night, when he returned to the hostel, he was obviously intoxicated and the staff would not let him in. He slept in the park for a while, but the police moved him on. He finally found a soup kitchen run by medical students at a nearby hospital. They gave him hot food and talked to him. One of the students strongly encouraged him to seek help and gave him the address of a night shelter. He went there, but it was full. The staff let him sleep in an outhouse and said that they would help him find a hostel space in the morning. By 6 am Sidney was experiencing withdrawal symptoms from alcohol. He was perspiring profusely and was tremulous. He felt anxious and panicky and was disorientated. He was not sure where he was or where he could get a drink from.

At 8 am one of the staff came in to see him and offered him an appointment with a Community Psychiatric Nurse (CPN), Ruth, who visited the shelter. Ruth was coming that day and could see him at 9 am. Sidney did not particularly want to see her, but he agreed. Ruth assessed Sidney's withdrawal symptoms and arranged for him to have a single dose of chlordiazepoxide (Librium) to reduce his withdrawal symptoms. She also arranged a bed for him in a nearby hostel, and said that she would visit him later that day. She visited him on a daily basis and managed a community detoxification over a week, using a reducing dose of chlordiazepoxide. The advice from the British National Formulary (BNF) is that parenteral thiamine should be given to all patients at risk of Wernike's encephalopathy (Joint Formulary Committee 2007). As Sidney did not have any symptoms of Wernike's encephalopathy or delirium tremens Ruth arranged for Sidney to take oral thiamine as a preventative measure. She also gave dietary advice.

Table 8.1   Suggested withdrawal regime

Day 1	20 mg chlordiazepoxide four times daily
Day 2	15 mg chlordiazepoxide four times daily
Day 3	10 mg chlordiazepoxide four times daily
Day 4	5 mg chlordiazepoxide four times daily
Day 5	5 mg chlordiazepoxide twice daily

Data taken from Parker *et al.* (2008)

Parker et al. (2008) suggest a withdrawal regime for community and in-patient settings in moderate dependence (see Table 8.1).

Severe dependence would require larger doses in an in-patient setting. Note that people experiencing delirium tremens or who are at high risk for seizures may need to be treated longer and must be admitted to hospital or a specialist residential facility with medical and emergency cover.

During the detoxification period Ruth gradually talked to Sidney about his past history and asked him if she could contact the hospitals in which he had been an in-patient to find out what his treatment had been. She arranged for him to see a psychiatrist, who said that he would reassess Sidney when he had been through the detoxification process and been abstinent for 2 weeks. Ruth explained the association between his alcoholism, homelessness and mental health problems to Sidney. He felt more able to accept the diagnoses and how they were interrelated. Ruth was part of a team that specialised in mental health problems in homeless people and also provided integrated treatment for dual diagnosis. If Sidney had been treated by a substance misuse agency, it is possible that his mental health problems would not have been addressed; and if he had been treated by mental health services, it is also possible that the implications of his alcohol dependence would not have been understood. There is the possibility that neither agency would have agreed to treat him, since the primary disorder would not have been clear at the assessment stage. Ruth was working in a specialist homeless team and so she did not have to adhere to rules about patient categories and could follow Sidney up, even when he moved addresses, or did not have an address; his treatment was therefore easily obtainable.

In her personal account of integrated treatment, Green (1996) describes how crucial education is in the treatment of the patient with dual diagnosis. Ruth needed to assess Sidney's perceptions about his two disorders because he could use his diagnosis of bipolar affective disorder as a reason to continue drinking, or alternatively focus only on being mentally ill, thus avoiding acceptance of the alcohol problem. Educating patients with dual diagnoses can be useful in preventing relapse (Daley 1986).

The psychiatrist returned to see Sidney after a 2-week period of abstinence and suggested that he should take fluoxetine (Prozac) and consider taking lithium carbonate again. He said that Ruth would monitor his lithium levels in the community and explained about the possible side-effects. The psychiatrist explained that the efficacy of the fluoxetine would be improved if Sidney did not drink.

Ruth implemented a care package that included a full physical examination including liver function tests, which were carried out at a medical centre for homeless people; she also employed relapse prevention techniques, helping Sidney to identify cues and triggers for his drinking. At the initial stages of recovery, she capitalised on the ambivalence he felt about his drinking and the effect it was having on his social functioning, employing motivational interviewing techniques. Ruth was aware of a transtheoretical model of change suggested by Prochaska and DiClemente (1984; 1998), which targets interventions towards the stage of change the individual is in relating to their substance use.

Ruth encouraged Sidney to spend time away from the hostel and helped him to enrol on a computer course, in order to structure his time and help him avoid other drinkers. This also had a beneficial effect on his self-esteem. She made an application to the local council citing Sidney's diagnosis of bipolar affective disorder as the reason he was in priority need. Housing is an important issue for people with dual diagnosis, as continuing homelessness is associated with a poor prognosis (Power & Attenborough 2003).

Ruth also recognised that Sidney used alcohol as a way of dealing with difficult feelings, in particular, those relating to the road traffic accident and his estrangement from his children and mother. Although cognitive therapy techniques can be useful at this stage of recovery and offer a degree of flexibility (Raistrick et al. 2006), Ruth referred Sidney for psychodynamic psychotherapy, because she felt that the longstanding nature of the problem, dating back to his unresolved childhood conflicts, implied that this would be more beneficial to him.

Sidney's mental state was stabilised with lithium carbonate and he continued to abstain from alcohol. He gained employment in a computer project established by his local mental health trust. He was granted a tenancy from the local authority following Ruth's application for housing. He started twice weekly psychodynamic psychotherapy 6 months after his detoxification programme. He continued to see Ruth weekly for 2 years.

Conclusion

This chapter and case study highlight some of the issues about alcohol and mood disorder. Although there is a lot of data about the aetiology of dual diagnosis emanating both from Europe and the United States, very little has been written about treatment strategies. Strategies described come from the author's own experience of working with people with dual diagnosis who are homeless.

References

Bakken K, Landheim AS, Valgum P (2003) Primary and secondary substance misusers: do they differ in substance-induced and substance independent mental disorders? *Alcohol and Alcoholism* 38: 54–59.

Beck A, Steer RA, Trexler LD (1989) Alcohol abuse and eventual suicide: a 5–10 year prospective study of alcohol abusing suicide attempters. *Journal of Studies on Alcohol* 50: 202–209.

Bhui K, Puffett A (1994) Sexual problems in the psychiatric and mentally handicapped populations. *British Journal of Hospital Medicine* 51: 459–464.

Borup C, Unden M (1994) Combined fluoxetine and disulfiram treatment of alcoholism with comorbid affective disorders: a naturalistic outcome study, including quality of life measurements. *European Psychiatry* 9: 83–89.

Bradwejn J, Jones BD, Annable L, Greese I, Choulnard A (1983) Neuroleptic blood levels. Proceedings of the Annual Meeting, Society of Biological Psychiatry, pg. 103 cited in Rubinstein L, Campbell F, Daley D (1990) *Four Perspectives on Dual Diagnosis: An Overview of Treatment Issues.* New Jersey: Howard Press Inc.

Brown GW, Harris T (1978) *Social origins of depression: a study of psychiatric disorder in women.* Abingdon: Taylor & Francis.

Ciraulo DA, Barnhill J (1988) Clinical pharmacokinetics of imipramine and desimipramine in alcoholics and normal volunteers. *Clinical Pharmacological Therapy* 509–518.

Cornelius JR, Salloum IM, Mezzich J, *et al.* (1995) Disproportionate suicidality in patients with comorbid major depression and alcoholism. *American Journal of Psychiatry* 152: 358–364.

Daley D (1986) *Relapse Prevention Workbook for Alcoholics and Drug Dependent Persons.* Florida: Learning Publications Inc.

Department of Health (2002) *Mental Health Policy Implementation Guide: Dual Diagnosis Good Practice Guide.* London: The Stationery Office.

Ericksen KP, Trocki KF (1994) Sex, alcohol and sexually transmitted diseases: a national survey. *Family Planning Perspectives* 26 (6): 257–263.

Gorman DM (1992) Distinguishing primary and secondary disorders in studies of alcohol dependence and depression. *Drug and Alcohol Review* 11 (1): 23–29.

Green VL (1996) The resurrection and the life. *American Journal of Orthopsychiatry* 66: 12–16.

Helzer JE, Pryzbeck TR (1988) The co-occurrence of alcoholism with other psychiatric disorders in the general population and its impact on treatment. *Journal of Studies on Alcohol* 49 (3): 219–224.

Holmes SJ, Robins LN (1987) The influence of childhood disciplinary experience on the development of alcoholism and depression. *Journal of Child Psychology and Psychiatry and Allied Disciplines* 28: 399–415.

Hussein Rassool GH (ed) (2006) *Dual Diagnosis Nursing*. Singapore: Blackwell Publishing Ltd.

Joint Formulary Committee (2007) *British National Formulary*, 54th Edition. London: British Medical Association and Royal Pharmaceutical Society of Great Britain.

Lamb H (1982) Young adult chronic patients: the new drifters. *Hospital and Community Psychiatry* 33: 465–468.

Madden JS (1994) Psychiatric syndromes associated with alcohol and substance misuse. In *Seminars in Alcohol and Drug Misuse*. London: Royal College of Psychiatrists.

O'Connel RA, Mayo JA, Flatow L (1991) Outcome of bi-polar disorder on long-term treatment with lithium. *British Journal of Psychiatry* 159: 123–129.

Parker A, Marshall EJ, Ball DM (2008) Diagnosis and management of alcohol user disorders. *British Medical Journal* 336: 496–501.

Power C, Attenborough J (2003) Up from the streets: a follow-up study of people referred to a specialist team for the homeless mentally ill. *Journal of Mental Health* 12 (1): 41–49.

Prime Minister's Strategy Unit (PMSU) (2004) *Alcohol Harm Reduction Strategy for England*. London: Cabinet Office.

Prochaska JO, DiClemente CC (1984) *The Transtheoretical Approach: Crossing the Boundaries of Therapy*. Illinois: Dow Jones-Irwin.

Prochaska JO, DiClemente CC (1998) Comments, criteria and creating better models in response to Davidson. In: Miller WR, Heather N (eds). *Treating Addictive Behaviors: Processes of Change*, 2nd Edition, pp. 39–45. New York: Plenum Press.

Raistrick D (2000) Management of alcohol detoxification. *Advances in Psychiatric Treatment* 6: 348–355.

Raistrick D, Heather N, Godfrey C (2006) *Review of the Effectiveness of Treatment for Alcohol Problems*. London: National Treatment Agency for Substance Misuse.

Roy A (1996) Aetiology of secondary depression in male alcoholics. *British Journal of Psychiatry* 169: 753–757.

Rubinstein L, Campbell F, Daley D (1990) Four perspectives on dual diagnosis: an overview of treatment issues. In: *Managing the Dually Diagnosed Patient*. New York: Haworth Press Inc.

Schover L (1988) *Sexuality and Chronic Illness: A Comprehensive Approach*. New York: Guildford Press.

Schuckit MA (1986) Genetic and clinical implications of alcoholism and affective disorder. *American Journal of Psychiatry* 143: 140–147.

Schuckit MA, Maristela G (1988) Alcoholism, anxiety and depression. *British Journal of Addiction* 83 (12): 1373–1380.

Schuckit MA, Tipp JE, Bergman M, Reich W, Hesselbrock VM, Smith TL (1997) Comparison of induced and independent major depressive disorders in 2,945 alcoholics. *American Journal of Psychiatry* 154: 948–957.

Steele CM, Josephs RA (1990) Alcohol myopia: its prized and dangerous effects. *American Psychologist* 45: 921–933.

Straus MA, Kantor GK (1994) Corporal punishment of adolescents by parents: a risk factor in the epidemiology of depression, suicide, alcohol abuse, child abuse and wife beating. *Adolescence* 29: 543–561.

Timms PW, Fry AH (1989) Homelessness and mental illness. *Health Trends* 21: 70–71.

Torrens M, Fonseca F, Mateu G, Farre M (2005) Efficacy of antidepressants in substance use disorders with and without comorbid depression. A systematic review and meta-analysis. *Drug and Alcohol Dependence* 78: 1–22.

Wasserman D, Varnik A, Eklund G (1994) Male suicides and alcohol consumption in the former USSR. *Acta Psychiatrica Scandinavica* 89: 306–313.

Chapter 9

Polysubstance Use and Personality Disorder

Simon McArdle

Introduction

There are increased rates of psychiatric disorders among those who have problematic substance use. Approximately one-third of heavy drinkers have associated mental health problems, and one-half of drug users have mental health problems. Such mental health problems result in increased rates of service utilisation, poorer levels of social functioning and, overall, appear to be associated with poorer outcome. Although drug and alcohol use per se do not constitute grounds for compulsory admission to hospital, patients may become so severely psychologically disturbed or suicidal as a result of using drugs that treatment is essential to protect themselves or others.

Prevalence

Personality disorders and substance use commonly co-occur, particularly with antisocial personality disorders (ASPD) and borderline personality disorders (BPD) (Moran *et al.* 2006). ASPD, BPD and substance use share a set of personality traits, particularly, impulsiveness and sensation seeking. Personality disorders and substance use are strongly associated with depression, which may exacerbate the severity of substance use and depressive symptoms.

Service delivery

In light of this context, service delivery is now focused on mainstream mental health services providing assessment, management and treatment of people with mental disorders and substance use disorders (DH 2002; NIMHE 2003). Mental health professionals in most settings are expected as part of the core proficiencies to be able to work at some level with people presenting with these issues. In view of this recent shift, this chapter is an attempt to provide practical guidance and support for such workers. Although much of the material used will be taken from the specialisms of substance use practice and personality disorder practice, the principles, roles and skills identified are core characteristics that can readily be adopted by mental health professionals in most contexts. The chapter will concentrate on key characteristics of the work and will provide recommendations for working with this client group. The key recommendations are that working with personality disorder and substance use disorder require comprehensive and rigorous assessment and structured treatment approaches. This said, mental health professionals work in many different settings, with different approaches to care, and it is acknowledged that there is no single way of working as a mental health professional (Coyne & Wright 1997: 23).

What is personality disorder?

Personality disorder is defined as a functional impairment or psychological distress resulting from inflexible and maladaptive personality traits. This impairment is demonstrated in thinking styles, affectivity, impulse control and, particularly, how the person relates to other people. The problem must then be persistent over time and pervasive across a variety of situations. Substance use problems are a defining criterion for some personality disorders (ASPD, BPD), and some personality disorder features can be directly or indirectly related to substance use, for example, irritability, irresponsibility and affective instability.

The Home Office estimates that there are approximately 250,000–300,000 problematic drug users in England who require treatment (National Treatment Agency [NTA] 2006a). The rate of substance misuse among the general population has been estimated at approximately 6%, while the rate of substance misuse among people with mental health problems is approximately one-third to a half (Regier *et al.* 1990). Overall evidence suggests that a significant proportion of patients in mental health service in-patient settings are drug or alcohol users (Phillips & Johnson 2003).

The literature on some aspects of personality disorder identifies an element of 'externalising spectrum' characterised by 'overt acting out and a general lack of behavioural control' (Taylor & Lang 2006). The clinical presentation of substance misuse and the two frequently co-morbid personality disorders – ASPD and BPD – can be viewed as being on this spectrum. This is captured in familiar descriptions:

People with borderline personality disorder display a pattern of instability of mood, self-image and interpersonal relationships. They exhibit extremes of idealisation and devaluation. Repeated, persistent suicidal threats, gestures and behaviour are common. Impulsive spending, unsafe sex, binge eating or substance misuse can be self-damaging. Clients may experience paranoid ideation and dissociative symptoms. They tend to use substances in chaotic and unpredictable, multiple drug ways.... People with antisocial personality disorder usually have a history of chronic antisocial behaviour that begins before age 15 and continues into adulthood. Clients demonstrate a pattern of impulsive, irresponsible, rebellious and reckless behaviour, as indicated by academic failure, poor job performance (if a job is held at all) and illegal activities. There is a diminished capacity for intimacy and clients experience dysphoria. They do not tolerate boredom well and feel victimised. Many people with antisocial personality disorder use substances in a polydrug fashion. (Kettles 2006)

Treatment and intervention approaches

The complex needs of this client group require multidisciplinary team working and inter-agency collaboration and working in partnerships (DH, SODH, WO, DHSSNI 1999). This approach necessitates shared working across, and between, potential barriers. The following factors are relevant to the treatment of substance misuse and responsible for the development of 'shared care'. Shared care is a rational model to improve service delivery: it aims to deliver a flexible service, utilising differing skills in the most effective manner. The focus is on the use of primary services first and foremost. The Care Programme Approach (CPA) readily sits within this philosophy. A person with both personality disorder and substance use disorder will present with complex needs and will require enhanced CPA status (DH 2006).

McMurran (2002a) observed that treatments for personality disorders per se tend to be broad-based, addressing a range of interpersonal behaviours, cognitions, attitudes, beliefs and emotional control. These broad-based programmes are usually group treatments, often residential, and while they may be principally cognitive behavioural, they often incorporate elements from other approaches, for instance, psychodynamic therapies or therapeutic communities. Because of these complexities, it is difficult to identify which are the key elements in treatment.

There is a wide range of effective treatments for substance misuse (Beaumont 2004). These include

- detoxification;
- maintenance prescription;
- antagonist prescription;
- therapeutic communities;
- motivational enhancement therapy;
- counselling and psychotherapy;

- cognitive behaviour therapies;
- family and relationship therapies;
- community reinforcement;
- combinations of the above.

There are a number of fundamental principles of effective treatment (Kettles 2006 citing National Institute on Drug Abuse 1999) review:

- No single treatment is appropriate for all individuals.
- Treatment needs to be readily available.
- Effective treatment attends to multiple needs of the individual, not just his or her drug use.
- An individual's treatment and services plan must be assessed continually and modified as necessary to ensure that the plan meets the person's changing needs.
- Remaining in treatment for an adequate period of time is critical for effective treatment (minimum 3 months).
- Counselling (individual or group) and other behavioural therapies are critical components of effective treatment for addiction.
- Medications are an important element of treatment for many patients, especially when combined with other behavioural therapies.
- Addicted or drug-using individuals with coexisting mental disorders should have both disorders treated in an integrated way.
- Medical detoxification is only the first stage of addiction treatment and by itself does little to change long-term drug use.
- Treatment does not have to be voluntary to be effective.
- Possible drug use during treatment must be monitored continuously.
- Treatment programmes should provide assessment for blood-borne viral illnesses, as well as counselling.
- Recovery from addiction is a long-term process and frequently requires multiple episodes of treatment.

Assessment

When working with people with personality disorder, it is necessary to undertake a comprehensive assessment (Bateman & Tyrer 2002; Craissati *et al.* 2002). Building on this assessment, the clinical team then needs to employ a structured treatment model. A consistent feature of the models of care for substance misuse is the need for comprehensive assessment (NTA 2006a, 2006b). Building on a thorough assessment, the NTA (2006a, 2006b) recommends the use of structured treatment models.

Management and treatment must be considered in the context of the natural history of drug use. Awareness of the different stages substance users pass through can help the clinician make the right responses. The natural history of most regular substance users is like that of the general population, with general reductions in consumption and increased cessation rates with age. There are many social pressures dissuading adults from ongoing drug use, and the social consequences of ongoing heavy drug use result in significant marginalisation of those who persist in use.

Stages of change

The stages of change model (Prochaska & DiClemente 1983) has important practical applications for assessment and treatment. Motivation is considered to be a precondition for treatment, and this model assists the clinician to encourage motivation. The model recognises that substance users engage in change when they have passed through various key stages. These key stages are precontemplation, contemplation, decision, action, maintenance and relapse.

- *Precontemplation:* There is no awareness that there is a problem.
- *Contemplation:* There is awareness that a problem exists and that change might be necessary. Persons begin to weigh up the pros and cons of their substance misuse; they feel somewhat ambivalent about their behaviour and about change.
- *Decision:* There is a point reached where a decision is made to do nothing or something.
- *Action:* This is the process or stage of doing something.
- *Maintenance:* The task is to consolidate and maintain the gains that have been achieved.
- *Relapse:* There is a return to previous patterns of behaviour at a contemplative stage. Importantly, relapse in itself is not considered a treatment failure but a positive learning experience, potentially increasing the successful outcome next time round.

The value of this model is that it clarifies which stage the individual substance user is at and this informs the clinical response. Clinical interventions must be tailored to match the client's needs at a given point in time.

Patients with coexisting substance use and mental health problems present many challenges. It is acknowledged that, as a group, patients with dual diagnosis are more difficult to manage and treat because of their complex needs. Patients with dual diagnosis tend to place a heavy demand on service provision and have been associated with poor outcomes on most measures – housing status, employment status, social functioning and family relationships.

The failure to recognise mental health problems among substance users, and vice versa, can lead to ineffective management and treatment outcomes. It is often difficult to distinguish between symptoms related to substance use and those related to mental illness. There are several possible explanations for the patient's condition. First, the patient's use might have developed against a background of an underlying disorder that predated substance use. Second, the patient's disorder might be related to the negative physical, social and psychological sequelae associated with substance use. Finally, a psychiatric disorder and a substance misuse disorder might occur independently of each other.

The task in assessing the needs of the patient is compounded by poor insight. This is further complicated by the fact that patients might use a combination of substances (polydrug use). Historically, health care services adopted a prescriptive position that to make an accurate assessment it is necessary for the patient to be drug-free for 4 to 6 weeks (Nathan 1991 cited in Rassool 2002). The reality of substance use problems and the contemporary clinical world are very different. Health care professionals have had to adopt a more realistic, flexible and proactive position in the context of high prevalence of substance use in mental health service settings.

The key message currently is that the assessment and management of substance use are core competences required by clinical staff in mental health services (DH 2006). The guidance aims

- to encourage integration of drug and alcohol expertise and related training into mental health service provision;
- to provide ideas and guidance to front-line staff and managers to help them provide the most effective therapeutic environments;
- to help mental health services plan action on dual diagnosis.

The National Service Framework for Mental Health (DH, SODH, WO, DHSSNI 1999) identifies patients with dual diagnosis as a population with a greater risk of stigmatisation and exclusion from existing service provision. Professionals might be reluctant to intervene with patients with dual diagnosis because of the lack of knowledge and expertise, or a negative attitude towards patients with dual diagnosis. Overtly self-destructive behaviour may be met with suppressive and moralistic responses by many professionals, possibly out of a sense of frustration or inadequacy about an ability to effect any change (Hussein Rassool 2002).

People with co-morbid personality disorder, particularly ASPD, are more likely to drop out of substance use treatment, but there is evidence that this may actually be related to co-morbid depression rather than personality disorder (Kokkevi *et al.* 1998 cited in McMurran 2002b). Since treatment completion is important to a good outcome, it is crucial to assess for, and treat depression in, substance users, with or without personality disorder, although it is worth bearing in mind that withdrawal from substances may actually be the cause of low mood. It is also essential to assess for, and treat where necessary, risk of self-harm and suicidality.

It is clear that substance use may interfere with the assessment of, treatment of and recovery from mental health problems. Individual assessments are likely to identify the need for 'simple interventions' for substance use rather than a need for specialist addiction skills. A substantial number of patients may respond to simple motivational interventions provided by mental health staff as part of the overall care plan (DH 2006). More severe or complex substance use will require specialist interventions. In these cases, integrated, joint or coordinated working with substance misuse services is likely to be required in the context of the CPA provision and 'shared care' philosophy mentioned earlier. Following a comprehensive assessment, a care plan should be agreed upon with the client. It should cover the client's need as identified in one or more of the following four key domains:

- Drug and alcohol use
- Physical and psychological health
- Criminal involvement and offending
- Social functioning (NTA 2006b)

Working with patients who use substances often raises a variety of concerns for mental health staff, in particular, worries about competence to deal with the issues, access to appropriate specialist services when needed and the legal and ethical implications of actions such as drug testing, searching service users and their belongings, discharging services users who do not adhere to boundaries and involving the police (DH 2006). The rest of this chapter will address some of these practical treatment and management issues.

The extent of current use and problems should be explored through initial screening questions. A number of simple questions can be useful:

- What substances is the individual using?
- In what quantities; how frequently?
- By what route?
- How long have they been using in this way?
- Do they see this use as problematic?
- Previous treatment episodes and outcomes?

This screening should include an examination of the following:

- General behaviour
- Mood

- Delusions and hallucinations
- Confusional states

Before any biological screening test, full informed consent should be obtained from the patient (DH, SODH, WO & DHSSNI 1999). In traditional treatment settings where consent is not given for such tests, discussion frequently focuses on discharge. It is helpful clinically if clients are encouraged to cooperate with testing. Where appropriate, routine or random testing needs to be incorporated in care plans and to be part of a whole treatment plan. Testing does, however, have a place where there is reason to think that self-reporting may not be accurate. A number of practical considerations may be useful, although those listed subsequently for obtaining urine samples is neither intended as a definitive list nor precludes the need to follow local documentation and to individualise care:

- Testing should occur on admission and randomly throughout treatment.
- Consent must be obtained on each occasion.
- Dip-testing must be done in the presence of the patient.
- Information about approximate drug detection times must be available.
- Clinical decisions must not be made on the basis of one positive test.
- Searching is important where there is a risk to the safety of the service user or other service users.
- Searching must be used with awareness that personal searches are a serious invasion of service users' privacy and rights.
- Consent should always be sought and the reasons for the search must be clearly explained and always the care planned.
- Searches must take place by and in the presence of the same gender staff.
- Consent under duress is not a valid consent.
- If there is evidence that drug dealing is occurring, then consideration should be given to seeking police assistance (in accordance with the outcomes of the 'Wintercomfort' case).

Where illicit substances are found, the following factors need to be considered (DH 2006):

- Contact local pharmacy if drugs from the pharmacy-controlled drugs stock are found as listed in Schedules 2, 3 and 4 of the Misuse of Drugs Regulations (2001).
- Contact local police if illegal drugs are found as listed in Schedule 1 of the Misuse of Drugs Regulations (2001).
- Illegal drugs that are not handed to the police should also be destroyed once it is determined they are no longer required.
- Non-prescribed drugs must also be destroyed as soon as possible once it is determined they are no longer required.

Section 5(4) of the Misuse of Drugs Act (1971 cited in DH 2006) provides a defence for hospital staff who take possession of patients' illegal drugs to protect a patient from harm or prevent another from committing a crime of unlawful possession or for the purpose of delivering it into lawful custody.

Substances that patients have held lawfully before admission cannot be destroyed without a service user's consent, and they have the right for such items to be returned to them at the time of their discharge. Wherever possible, however, service users should be encouraged to allow staff to dispose of substances such as prescribed controlled drugs or alcohol. Consent should be obtained in writing.

The assessment phase should also include observing for psychiatric symptoms relating to intoxication or withdrawal from various psychoactive substances (DH 2006).

A good assessment will assist the nurse and the client to clarify how the person got to his or her present situation and where and how he or she wants to change (Clancy & Coyne 1997 cited in Coyne & Wright 1997: 32). This is essential to the work and needs to be established at the outset of the working relationship. This clarity will further help in the next stage of boundary setting. The ability to work with boundaries is crucial to the participation of both nurse and patient when working with complex needs. Unacceptable behaviour on the part of the client needs a clear, calm and precise response at the level of the individual nurse, the nursing team working at that time, the multidisciplinary team (MDT) as a whole and the service also. Clear, therapeutic boundaries, fairly and firmly implemented, will help clients to feel respected, confident and safe.

Realistic treatment goals need to be set and reviewed on a frequent and regular basis (DH 2006: 11–12). The targets may include any of the following:

- Initial focus on reducing the harm caused by substance misuse
- Stabilisation of drug use by prescribing a substitute mostly
- Detoxification/assisted withdrawal

Where a patient is involved in the misuse of substances a number of factors need to be considered. Factors that will need to be taken into account include

- seriousness and extent of the problem, including any legal issues;
- patient's mental state;
- risk of harm to self and others;
- patient's social circumstances;
- input from relatives and carers;
- patient's fitness for discharge;
- appropriate action if the patient repeats the use of illegal drugs;
- intensity of observation and supervision arrangements;

- reviewing leave arrangements;
- possibility and usefulness of transfer to another ward/setting;
- possibility of contacting the police;
- potential for prosecution or other sanctions.

Treatment plans and discharge arrangements for patients with substance misuse need to take account of relapse prevention. Relatives and carers should, where appropriate, be involved in these arrangements. There needs to be rapid follow-up arrangements in place as part of the CPA. This group tends to be at high risk of deterioration of mental state and can be at an increased risk of suicide or of violence to others. For those who have undergone detoxification from heroin while being an in-patient, there is an increased risk of overdose shortly after discharge. For severe and complex cases and when service users are willing to be referred, referral to specialist drug and alcohol services should be considered and should usually take place prior to discharge.

Arrangements for discharge for non-completers of treatment and premature leavers should still aim to provide an integrated plan. While an episode or programme of nursing care needs to be formally opened, so too does the closing of the work (Saunders 1986 cited in Coyne & Wright 1997: 42). This is no more important in premature discharge or discharge of non-completers. A patient may walk out of treatment or be prematurely discharged by the MDT as part of the care planned and contracted response to mutually agreed exclusion/discharge criteria. The ability to work with the frustrations and anxieties of these situations is an essential part of the skill-set for the individual nurse, nursing team on duty, MDT as a whole and the service itself, if it is in the business of working with complex needs.

Even in the midst of chaos and making the necessary compromise with that chaos which is central to the work (Cox 1978), it is contingent on all levels that the discharge of the non-completer or premature leaver is not a complete and utter surprise and something about which there is full and considered thought and reflection as it happens. When we are in the work and in the midst of the anxiety of working with complex needs at chaotic times, we need a simple and basic containing process:

- Infringements need to be managed immediately, both verbally and in writing.
- Team working is of particular importance under such circumstances.
- Warnings and the consequences of a warning being issued must be clear.
- Discharges should be respectful and assertive.
- Opportunities to re-engage should be made explicit.
- Successes need to be listed and made explicit.
- Take a fair, assertive and firm approach.
- Do not take an angry, tardy and disorganised approach.

- 'Splitting'on the clients' part can make these situations dangerous.
- Poor understanding of the aggression and violence policy on the staff's part can make these situations dangerous (Coyne & Wright 1997).

All of this approach is predicated on one key characteristic of treatment regardless of model–the ability of staff to work with therapeutic boundaries with patients who constantly test and violate boundaries. All nursing interventions for boundary maintenance should have as one basic aim the decrease in treatment resistance and increase in motivation (Schafer 2002). The challenge for nursing staff is that the patient's resistance and motivation cannot be dismissed as a part of the patient's pathology alone, but must be understood in the context of the therapeutic relationship (Miller & Rollnick 1991). The behaviour we are describing is one which can prompt nurses to have a sense of failure rather than progress both in relation to the patient and themselves. There can be a sense of management rather than treatment and of disengagement, staff may be pulled into engaging in power struggles with patients or withdraw because of patient's hostility and abuse and criticism of them as people (Main 1989; Schafer 2002).

Therapeutic principles

There are a number of fundamental principles, roles and skills for mental health nursing when working with people with personality disorder and substance misuse disorder. In a comprehensive review of *Forensic Mental Health Nursing* with such patients, Kettles (2006: 183–185) identifies a number of principles, skills and roles for forensic mental health nurses. 'I would argue that all mental health nurses in all contexts need to share these, and quote the principles which are crucial to this work by way of recommendation to colleagues and conclusion':

- There is a need to engage in a therapeutic nurse–patient relationship with **trust** as the foundation of the relationship and **clarity** in the goal, purpose and direction of the relationship.
- Appropriate **limit setting** is essential.
- The person requires assistance with the first phase of the treatment programme: **detoxification**.
- There is a need to recognise and avoid/deal with **power struggles** and/or withdrawal.
- The nurse needs to recognise and obtain help with **distorted forms of caring** and to avoid **splitting**.
- Develop an appropriate **treatment programme** that includes aspects of both personality disorder and substance misuse/management in an integrated manner.

- Other health professionals need to be **engaged** with the treatment programme.
- **Maintain** the **relationship** as it moves fully into the second phase of the treatment programme (remember this is a long-term process).
- Provide **relationship disengagement** at the appropriate time.
- Enable social support mechanisms and other **support mechanisms** for both yourself and the patient throughout and after the treatment programme.

Conclusion

This chapter has sought to identify the main constructs around dual diagnosis and personality disorders and has reviewed a series of assessment and intervention strategies appropriate to this context.

References

Bateman A, Tyrer P (2002) Effective management of personality disorder. http://www.nimhe.org.uk/downloads/Bateman_Tyrer.doc

Beaumont B (2004) *Care of Drug Users in General Practice: A Harm Reduction Approach*. Oxford: Radcliffe Publishing.

Cox M (1978) *Structuring the Therapeutic Process: Compromise With Chaos*. London: Pergamon Press.

Coyne P, Wright S (1997) *Substance Use: Guidance on Good Clinical Practice for Specialist Nurses Working with Alcohol and Drug Users*. London: The Association of Nurses in Substance Abuse (ANSA).

Craissati J, Horne L, Taylor R (2002) Effective treatment models for personality disordered offenders. http://www.dh.uk/prod_consum_dh

DH, SODH, WO, DHSSNI (1999) *Drug Misuse and Dependence – Guidelines on Clinical Management*. London: HMSO.

DH (2002) *Mental Health Policy Implementation Guide. Dual Diagnosis Good Practice Guide*. London: HMSO.

DH (2006) *Dual Diagnosis in Mental Health Inpatient and Day Hospital Settings. Guidance on the Assessment and Management of Patients in Mental Health Inpatient and Day Hospital Settings Who have Mental Ill-health and Substance Use Problems*. London: DH.

Hussein Rassool G (2002) Substance misuse and mental health: an overview. *Nursing Standard* 16: 46–52.

Kettles AM (2006) Dual diagnosis of personality disorder and substance misuse. In: National Forensic Nurses' Research and Development Group (Ed) *Forensic Mental Health Nursing. Interventions with People with 'Personality Disorder'*. London: Quay Books.

Main T (1989) *The Ailment and Other Psychoanalytic Essays*. London: Free Association.

McMurran M (2002a) *Expert Paper: Personality Disorders*. Liverpool: National R&D Programme on Forensic Mental Health.

McMurran M (2002b) *Expert Paper: Dual Diagnosis of Mental Disorder and Substance Misuse*. Liverpool: National R&D Programme on Forensic Mental Health.

Miller WR, Rollnick S (1991) *Motivational Interviewing: Preparing People for Change in Addictive Behaviours*. London: Guilford.

Moran P, Coffey C, Mann A, Carlin JB, Patton GC (2006) Personality and substance use disorder in young adults. *British Journal of Psychiatry* 188: 374–379.

NIMHE (2003) *Personality Disorder: No Longer a Diagnosis of Exclusion*. London: DH.

National Treatment Agency for Substance Misuse (2006a) *Models of Care for Treatment of Adult Drug Misusers*. London: NTA. Update 2006.

National Treatment Agency for Substance Misuse (2006b) *Care Planning Practice Guide*. London: NTA.

Phillips P, Johnson S (2003) Drug and alcohol misuse among inpatients with psychotic illness in three inner London psychiatric units. *Psychiatric Bulletin* 27: 217–220.

Prochaska J, DiClemente C (1983) Stages and processes of self change of smoking, and towards a more integrative model of change. *Journal of Consulting and Clinical Psychology* 51: 390–395.

Regier D, Farmer M, Rae D (1990) Co-morbidity of mental disorders with alcohol and other drugs of abuse: results from the epidemiological catchment area. *Journal of the American Medical Association* 264: 2511–2518.

Schafer PE (2002) Nursing interventions and future directions with patients who constantly break rules and test boundaries. In: Kettles AM, Woods P, Collins M (Eds). *Therapeutic Interventions for Forensic Mental Health Nurses*. London: Jessica Kingsley.

Taylor J, Lang AR (2006) Psychopathy and substance use disorders. In: CJ Patrick (Ed). *Handbook of Psychopathy*. New York: Guilford.

Chapter 10

Older People and Dual Diagnosis

Sue Excell

Introduction

Older people are frequently an overlooked population in the field of dual diagnosis. There is a public and media perception that such comorbidities relate mainly to the younger age population and this is a view that has been well documented by Deblinger (2000). Far more is known and publicly reported about dual diagnosis in adults below the age of 60; for example, younger adults who attract much attention in media reports for excessive binge drinking, which has been closely linked to an increase in violent assaults and antisocial behaviour. However, the author's experience of working within mental health services for older people is that dual diagnosis among older people has become more of a pressing issue.

This chapter examines the impact of dual diagnosis on older adults, exploring the key issues that arise in relation to this, including the following:

- Media representation of facts on alcohol use
- Policy and strategic framework
- Reporting and diagnosis
- The meaning of old age
- Over-the-counter (OTC) and prescription medication
- Conclusion
- Case studies

An increasing population

Older people are the fastest growing population to cause 'significant health concern'; O'Connell (2003) refers to this as 'an impending demographic time bomb'. During the late nineteenth century much of the world experienced a process called 'demographic transition', which gave rise to the relatively large older population that is seen in the United Kingdom and much of the world today. The group aged 80 and above is by far the fastest growing group in the older population. The significant increase in the numbers of this group, coupled with their diverse health and social care needs, will present many challenges for the provision of health and for social care providers for the future.

The generation that is most likely to be associated with the significant increase in illicit drug and alcohol abuse are the 'baby boomers', a cohort born in the two decades following World War II (1945–1965) who are now approaching what is considered 'old age', their sixties. The baby boomers are cohorts who have lived within an environment that has widely accepted and encouraged the use of alcohol, as it has become more available, cheaper and less controlled. Larger numbers of current users are expected to continue their habit as they reach 65 years (Patterson & Jeste 1999). A significant increase in demand on health and social care services can be anticipated. Other authors such as Phillips and Katz (2001) identify that older people with a dual diagnosis are one of the most neglected areas in terms of service provision and empirical research.

Policy framework

The National Service Framework for Older People (2001) reports that between 1995 and 2025 the number of people in the United Kingdom above the age of 80 is set to increase by half, and those over 90 years will double. Examples of national policy that inform the subject area are found in the *Dual Diagnosis Good Practice Guide* (Department of Health 2002) where 'mainstreaming' of dual diagnosis patients is seen as essential to providing effective care for complex clients, avoiding patients experiencing being 'shunted' between services. The policy refers to specific groups of people, for example, men, women, and adolescents. However, older adults appear to have been excluded from the overall discussion, noted as an 'identified service shortfall' without discussion or debate as to how best to meet the needs of this growing population.

Other recent policy directives that have been introduced by the government have traditionally been concentrated on the needs of younger people; they consider the prevention of illicit drug use and the link between drugs, alcohol and crime (Cabinet Office 2000). At present, within the United Kingdom attitudes to the policing and supply of drugs are scaled according to their classification under the Drug Misuse Act 1971. Drugs are segregated into three classes, A, B and C, which indicate the level of danger with each drug, A class being the most harmful. Although currently there is an awareness of potentially rapidly accelerating harm from alcohol, it remains an unclassified drug and as such limits the opportunity to regard it as a harmful substance, and therefore it will continue to be ill defined (Nutt 2007).

As such, in the United Kingdom drugs and younger people have dominated the substance misuse policy agenda. Since older adults are not part of the government's drug use strategy, there remains a paucity of research literature relating to the issue (Phillips & Katz 2001). None of the national strategies, i.e. National Service Framework for Older People (2001) and National Alcohol Strategy, have taken the needs of older people seriously, if indeed they have considered it at all. First, there needs to be an understanding of the 'problem' in order that policy statements can be seen as taking the most appropriate action to ensure best practice. Lack of a clear commissioning framework and policy guidance in relation to developing specialist services for older people has had a negative impact on this invisible group, and has seriously disadvantaged an opportunity for empirical research and professional training in this much needed area.

However, for the first time the Department of Health will support service and financial mapping for specialist older people's mental health services. *Everybody's Business* (Department of Health 2005) describes a whole systems approach to commissioning integrated services, describing a shift in the role of the Primary Care Trusts towards promoting health across the whole of life. For older people, physical health and mental health are inextricably linked. This policy will be a key driver in eradicating discrimination on the basis of age and frailty. Health promotion must be seen as a continuum that addresses maintaining positive health, prevention, treatment and recovery throughout an all-age life cycle.

Media representation of information on alcohol

Alcohol-related issues are frequently reported through the media, which often lead to conflicting information on whether alcohol is seen as a positive or harmful effect on well-being. The following examples have been extracted from newspaper reports publicised between the years of 2002 and 2008. All articles relate to alcohol and older people's mental health issues. The author aims to establish that it is often media representation of information that coveys a mixed message to older people, leaving them struggling to understand what is meant by 'sensible' or 'safe' drinking and the impact moderate drinking has on physical and mental health well-being.

Hall (2002) reported that those who drink between one and three alcoholic drinks a day can reduce their risk of dementia in later life by 70%. Dutch researchers reported that light to moderate drinking reduced the risk of all types of dementia by 42%, concluding that 'a bit of what you fancy does you good'. Day (2004) reported that red wine in 'moderation' can have positive health benefits and that growing numbers of pensioners are binge-drinking at home. Both reports conclude that health promotion advice to encourage 'safe limits' is a key recommendation. Solfrizzi and Panza (2007) stated that one alcoholic drink a day can delay dementia in older people with mild memory loss, reporting that in total 121 people were monitored for $3^{1}/_{2}$ years, those who drank one glass of wine a day developed dementia at a rate that is 85% slower than for those who abstained.

Gilhooly (2007) reports that drinking guidelines should be introduced to protect the health of consumers and refers to the cohort of baby boomers who are more likely to drink excessively into old age, further reporting that older people should be advised not to drink at all, and should be aware of the effect alcohol has on their metabolism. Highfield (2008) alleged that drinking alcohol accelerates onset of Alzheimer's disease 5 years earlier than in those who do not drink.

Articles such as these demonstrate how easy it can be for people of any age to become confused or feel overwhelmed regarding the latest research or health promotion report. For most people, it is about enabling them to consider choices around lifestyle.

Perception of old age

What is meant by old age?

The question of what constitutes old age is a vexing one. It is arguable that this is not a purely academic debate as the central rationale for this subject is dual diagnosis and older people, positing the argument that in some way their needs differ from those of a younger person. What about the needs of a 70-year-old compared to the needs of an 89-year-old? Retirement has frequently been heralded as the onset of old age, with the introduction of the state pension in 1946, based on chronological age alone. This arbitrary age barrier is often seen as a benchmark to old age in both health and social care settings, and as such is seen as the transitory age at which people are automatically referred into older adult services. With people retiring earlier, the entire retired population will span over four decades, and as such cannot be referred to collectively as 'the retired' (Reed & Stanley 2004).

It may be more appropriate to reconsider old age in the context of dual diagnosis in that their physiological age is likely to be modified by virtue of their dual diagnosis per se. This generation is likely to present to services with a range of complex health and psycho-social concerns different from that of younger adults. All these issues will need to be addressed in UK national drug strategies and health policy provision.

Alcohol use in older people

There is far more research publicised on alcohol misuse in older people than drug misuse. This is largely because alcohol as a substance is more accessible and acceptable to older people. However, there are still fewer studies in this ageing population, compared to studies undertaken with younger people. People over 65 years commonly drink alcohol. Atkinson (1994) reports that the 1994 General Household Survey indicates that 17% of men and 7% of women above the age of 65 were exceeding 'sensible limits;' Jones and Joseph (1997) estimate that between 1 and 12% misuse it or have been identified as 'problem drinkers'. Other studies, Hartford and Samorajski (1982), Blazer and Pennybacker (1984), Ewing (1984), Atkinson (1991) and Adams *et al.* (1992), quote between 6 and 14% (heavy use) and between 1 and 17% (problematic use). The consensus in the literature is that the scale of the problem is far greater than what current measures suggest.

There is strong evidence to suggest that women above the age of 65 drink less than older men of a similar age. International studies as demonstrated by Mishra and Kastenbaum (1980) that in the United States women above the age of 65 are more likely to drink less than their male counterparts; this is further reiterated by Neve (1993) who reports that in the Netherlands women are more likely to abstain as they get older. Essentially two patterns of drinking have been described in older people, as being of early or late onset.

Older people who fall in the early-onset category have traditionally experienced a lifelong pattern of problem drinking and have probably been alcoholics most of their lives (Menninger 2002). They are more likely to experience mental health problems and organ brain syndromes. Studies from the United States state that this category comprises of two-thirds of older alcoholics (Gulino & Kadin 1986; Atkinson *et al.* 1990). About one-third of older people fall into the late-onset category. This group tends to be highly educated, and a stressful life event or emotional crisis precipitates or exacerbates their drinking. Brennan and Moos (1996) reported that in contrast to the early-onset drinkers, those in the late-onset category typically have fewer physical and mental health problems. Both these groups of people frequently fail to acknowledge their alcohol misuse and often drink secretly (Phillips & Katz 2001).

Complications of excessive alcohol use

Excessive alcohol use in older people can cause a wide range of physiological, physical and psychological problems, as well as increase the risk of coronary heart disease, hypertension and stroke (Department of Health 1995). Alcohol adds to the risks of accidents and is reported to be one of the three main reasons for falls (Wright & Whyley 1994). Alcohol may exacerbate Parkinson's disease in older people, and delirium tremens is associated with higher mortality rates in the older adult age group (Feuerlein & Reiser 1986). A particular concern is that older drinkers may mix alcohol with prescribed and OTC medication. It is reported that 8 out of 10 people aged 65 and older regularly take prescribed medication, one-third of people taking four or more prescribed drugs a day. Thus, there is a greater possibility of interactions with prescribed medication (Dunne 1994).

Assessment and screening

A further barrier to highlighting prevalence is the diagnostic criterion that has been developed for the younger age group and as such may not be valid and tested in an ageing population. The CAGE questionnaire, for example (Ewing 1984), is a widely used screening tool, but does not have high validity with older people, in particular, older women (Adams *et al.* 1996). However, some tools are more appropriate for older people, such as the Michigan Alcohol Screening Test, MAST-G (Blow *et al.* 1991), which has a high specificity and sensitivity with older people in a range of health care settings. The picture emerging from the literature remains confusing because of a lack of what is defined as an alcohol problem and the ranges of terminology that support it. Therefore, any review of the literature needs to interpret the literature to accommodate the varying definitions that are commonly used.

Under-reporting

There is an abundance of evidence to suggest that alcohol misuse is under-recognised and under-detected in this ageing population, for example Blazer and Pennybacker (1984), Curtis (1989), Dunne (1994), as few inquiries are made about this problem. Families, carers and professionals often deny any alcohol-related issues. This can be linked to the stigma attached to admitting a problem, or may be because the attitude of a person or professional deems that there is little point in attempting to change these behaviours. Dunne (1994) and Naik and Jones (1994) take this view one step further and report that even if older people are found to have an alcohol problem, it tends not to be adequately assessed or managed.

Over-the-counter medication (OTC)

Alcohol misuse in older people is not the only substance misused by older people. Misuse of OTC is frequently viewed as cheap, more accessible and relatively harmless (mistakenly) by older people. Kofoed (1985) reports that 10% of the general population regularly uses OTC medication compared to 69% of older people. It is, however, the authors' view that this is just as much if not more of a public health concern as alcohol misuse and is increasingly associated with chronic illnesses, such as heart disease, diabetes and arthritis.

Chronic illness such as these will be the challenge of the twenty-first century, as they already feature strongly in general practitioner (GP) consultations and in hospital admissions will be the challenge of the twenty first century, as they already feature strongly in general practitioner consultations and in hospital admissions. The author would suggest that as the care of older people becomes more community focused and increased demand placed on primary care, the role of the high street pharmacy will become crucial.

In addition, every year it is estimated that over 400,000 older people present to accident and emergency (A&E) departments following falls (Swift 2001). Poly-pharmacy is reported to be a major risk factor in the increase in falls in the above 65-year cohort of people. Older people are reported to use prescription medication three times more frequently than those of other age groups (Patterson & Jeste 1999).

The term misuse and abuse are frequently used in literature synonymously and are individually defined as 'to use to bad effect' (abuse) and to 'use wrongly' or 'apply wrong purpose' (misuse). The latter is felt by the author to be more pertinent as frequently older people are unaware that they are considered to be misusing their medication. Classes of drugs possibly misused in OTC include laxatives, antihistamines and alcohol-based liquid medication.

It is often difficult to establish misuse of medication, either OTC or prescribed, as frequently patients can present with a range of symptoms including the following:

- Sudden mood changes
- Irritability
- Poor concentration
- Acute confusional state
- Short-term memory loss

Prescribed medication

Benzodiazepines

Older adults receive more prescribed medication than the younger population in the United Kingdom. Morgan (1988) reports that this equates to 25% of all prescriptions, and of this percentage older people are far more likely to be prescribed benzodiazepines on long-term prescriptions. This 'medical' use of benzodiazepines, analgesics and hypnotics and other dependence-creating pharmaceuticals is often related directly to the ageing process and increased physical morbidity (Phillips & Katz 2001). Examples of this include analgesia for arthritis and benzodiazepines for bereavement, anxiety and insomnia. Typically, populations of older people in nursing and residential care environments receive a high proportion of psychoactive medication of a sedative nature (Ghodse 1997). Benzodiazepines may exacerbate a dementia process or cause misdiagnosis of what is referred to as 'iatrogenic pseudo dementia' (Closser 1991). According to Swartz *et al.* (1991), a predictive factor for benzodiazepine misuse is being 'old'.

Being aware that both prescription and OTC medication can be misused and be presented to professionals with other symptomatology presents an opportunity for clinicians to

- take a detailed drug history of OTC and other prescribed medication, including herbal and alternative therapy treatments;
- liaise with GP and family to take full history including any previous drug dependencies;
- use appropriate assessment and screening tools (Bartels *et al.* 2006).

The following case studies reflect working practices of the author; names have been altered and some details have been omitted.

CASE STUDY 1 (EARLY-ONSET DRINKING)

Ted is 76 years of age, married and lives with his wife. Ted is an early-onset drinker whose drinking history spans over 50 years. At the age of 16, he joined the army and with this he became part of the drinking culture that is still reported to be the norm today. He was previously known to the mental health service since experiencing episodes of depression as early as 1960.

The assessment

Ted had attempted to end his own life by taking an overdose; his circumstances leading to his admission were a noted deterioration in his mood and raised anxiety over a 6-month period. Ted had lost his son 5 years previously when he committed suicide; it was Ted who had found him. He had still not come to terms with his son's death and felt responsible as his son was also alcohol dependant. Ted had begun to isolate himself and his mood and dark thoughts had got progressively worse.

On admission to the acute ward Ted remained a suicide risk, and his wife reported violence towards her when he had been drinking. He had twice threatened her with a knife and on each occasion could not remember doing so. Ted was experiencing alcohol withdrawal symptoms and had a severe chest infection; he was also a heavy smoker. On a 'bad' day Ted would consume a bottle of whiskey and half a bottle of gin. He drank from early morning to late evening, when his aggression would be at its worst. His wife reported concerns over his deteriorating memory and his ability to drive without risk. She reported that for much of their married life she has had to be the stronger person in their relationship in order to cope with the children, manage their finances and support Ted through his heavy drinking patterns and episodes of depression. This has had a negative impact on their relationship, which is often strained and fraught with arguments over his chosen lifestyle.

The plan

Ted was transferred to the mental health unit and was placed on a detoxification programme and his withdrawal symptoms were closely monitored. A full alcohol screening and mental health history were obtained over a 3-week period. An in-depth risk assessment was also undertaken. Ted had a cognitive impairment and on a Mini Mental State Examination (MMSE) scored 18 out of 30. His formal diagnosis was mixed dementia with alcohol dependency.

Ted made good progress on the unit and soon gained weight. He had stopped smoking while being an in-patient and could now cycle several miles on an exercise bike. Following discharge, a plan to support him weekly in the community was agreed upon. Ted remained abstinent from alcohol for a period of 10 months with weekly follow-up and was introduced to a support group to promote his mental health and well-being. His cognitive status had improved to reveal an MMSE score of 24.

However, Ted then began to drink excessive cups of coffee (12 cups a day); caffeine is probably the most widely available stimulant and is present in a range of commercially available beverages including tea, coffee, and cola. Caffeine is frequently used by patients with mental health illness and can exacerbate psychotic symptoms and make them difficult to treat. Ted reported side effects including anxiety, poor concentration, disturbed sleep and tremors. A plan was put into place to decrease the use of caffeine over a 2-week period and replace his fluid intake with fruit juice and water. Ted then introduced decaffeinated coffee into his diet.

Following an unplanned home visit, Ted revealed that he had begun excessive drinking again, precipitated by acute pain following a fall. His mood was low and he had not taken any antidepressant medication for more than a week. A variety of pills had been stored in a pot in his room with intent to end his life. An emergency admission was agreed on; on further assessment Ted had a chest infection, had not eaten for 3 days and reported that the acute pain had reduced his quality of life significantly.

The admission lasted for 2 weeks on an informal basis, when Ted asked to be discharged. He has since had a further emergency admission following relapse. It has been 3 months since his discharge, his mood is improving, but his physical health and acute pain limit his quality of life. Ted has a pain management plan written by the GP and is slowly coming to terms with his failing physical ill health. Education has been provided to the primary care sector on alcohol and drug misuse in older people, as Ted had been prescribed a liquid morphine compound by his GP, which he became addicted to, and had begun to misuse. Since jointly working with the GP practice, prescribing has been reviewed more frequently, and better communication has enabled us jointly to manage his care.

The outcome

Although Ted has maintained complete abstinence from alcohol he continues to smoke excessively, and has no desire to stop. He is currently prescribed pain relief that is less addictive and reviewed in clinic monthly. Ted has good insight into his difficulties and recognises that his addictive behaviour has had a major impact on his quality of life.

CASE STUDY 2 (LATE-ONSET DRINKING)

Mary is a 71-year-old woman who is widowed and lives alone and is described as a late on-set drinker. She was referred to the older adult mental health service following an episode of depression and alcohol dependency. She had no previous mental health history. Her husband had been killed tragically in a road traffic accident only 6 months after they both retired. Mary and her husband had owned a restaurant and were looking forward to a planned retirement.

Mary had always enjoyed the company of others; the culture of this trade meant social drinking was part of the norm. Mary had begun excessive drinking shortly after her husband's death and was raw with grief and anger. She had not had an opportunity to say goodbye to her husband, and all their plans had now become a distant memory.

From the first initial meeting with her it was clear that her low mood and loss of appetite had contributed to significant weight loss, and through excessive drinking her appearance had begun to change, she had skin changes to her nose and face and her arms were badly bruised through endless falls. Her appearance was unkempt and her breath smelt strongly of stale alcohol. She had not eaten for 3 days and reported retching continuously with nothing but bile leaving her stomach.

The assessment

The first assessment using the Care Programme Approach was an opportunity to assess her physical and mental health status; liver function tests were undertaken and an anxiety and depression scale revealed that her mood was significantly low, with active thoughts of suicide. Mary was embarrassed about her drinking, experiencing feelings of guilt and shame that she had not only let herself down but her close family too. Time in the initial assessment was spent building a rapport and searching for something positive for Mary to hold onto. During this assessment motivational interviewing skills were utilised. Mary was stuck in the grieving process and could not see a fulfilling life alone. She described feeling a desperate need to cry and express emotion but every time it came close, the tears could not flow. It was evident throughout the assessment that she was experiencing withdrawal symptoms, as her hands were shaking continuously and her mouth was very dry.

Through the darkest days, Mary reported drinking 1–2 bottles of wine a day and then drank a litre of whisky every other day, usually at night. She identified this as her lowest point in the day, when it felt better to blot out the unhappy thoughts of loneliness and she thought the alcohol would help her sleep. This made her feel worse and often resulted in her falling, and waking up having slumped in a chair with no recollection of how she got there. Mary did not like the person she had become, and appeared relieved to have an opportunity to share her despair. The initial assessment ended on a positive note, which was that Mary was determined to accept help and promote opportunity for recovery.

The plan

Mary was offered and accepted an informal in-patient admission for detoxification, followed by a period of grief counselling. Detoxification took place over a period of 2 weeks and was successful; an anti-craving drug Acamprosate was prescribed, with positive effect. Mary participated in grief counselling, which commenced 4 weeks after discharge, for a period of 12 months. A planned community home visit was provided at the end of each week for 1 hour to review the medication and undertake motivational enhancement therapy (Miller & Rollnick 1991) to help achieve her goal of recovery. Mary decided after 3 months of complete abstinence that this was an unachievable goal, and has since chosen to stop Acamprosate. Mary still experiences occasions when excessive drinking takes over, usually precipitated by a stressful and anxiety-provoking situation. These occasions are far less frequent, and Mary has developed new coping strategies in order to help her overcome the embarrassment and guilt of her actions. She now recognises that too much stress is a trigger for increase in anxiety and that drinking alcohol can lead her down a path that she does not wish to go. Mary now phones and says she has had a bad day and talks through the situation, thus preventing prolonged periods of drinking.

The outcome

After close community working for 1 year, Mary looks and states she feels 10 years younger. Her skin has vastly improved and her physical health has improved too. Her dietary needs are met and she has gained weight. Her depression has lifted and she can now talk about the life she shared with her husband without feeling angry and distressed. Mary has sought a voluntary work placement with support to work with pre-school children, something she enjoyed doing previously in her life before having her own family. Mary shared a view that she always assumed that it was mainly men or younger people who misused alcohol, and now feels she can help others understand that it can happen to anyone, at any stage in life. Mary will co-facilitate dual diagnosis basic awareness workshops as part of a service initiative. She hopes to help staff understand the stigma attached to admitting a problem, and how being supported and empowered to make her own decisions and choices has helped her overcome a difficult part of her life, towards recovery.

Conclusion

Drug and alcohol misuse in older people is a complex, multi-factorial and not fully understood phenomenon. In contrast to the younger adult population older people are more likely to misuse OTC medication, prescribed drugs and alcohol, initiated because of increased physical, psychological and physiological morbidity. These issues make accurate measurement of the full extent of the problem extremely difficult to establish. National policy relating to the needs of older people and drug misuse remains rather vague, unchanged or unchallenged; this is largely due to the uncertainty or 'hidden' extent of older adult drug and alcohol problems and the lack of empirical evidence and evaluation to support effectiveness in the identification, assessment and treatment of the older person. It is therefore likely that drug and alcohol problems in older people are currently underestimated. Further research into the epidemiology and circumstances in which drug and alcohol misuse occur in older people needs to be a key priority at both a national and local health service level, this will ensure that appropriate and acceptable treatment programmes and services are developed that are based on need as opposed to age.

References

Adams WL, Barry KL, Flemming MF (1996) Screening for problem drinking in older primary care patients. *Journal of American Medical Association* 276: 1964–1967.

Adams WL, Magruder-Habib K, Trued S, *et al.* (1992) Alcohol abuse in elderly emergency department patients. *Journal of the American Geriatric Society* 40: 1236–1240.

Atkinson RM (1990) Ageing and alcohol use disorders, diagnostic issues in the elderly. *International Psychogeriatric Journal* 2 (1): 55–72.

Atkinson RM (1991) Alcohol and drug abuse in the elderly. In: Jacoby R, Oppenheimer C (eds). *Psychiatry in the Elderly.* Oxford: Oxford Medical Publication.

Atkinson RM (1994) *General Household Survey.* London: Her Majesty Stationary Office.

Bartels S, Blow FC, Ban Critters AD, Brockman LM (2006) Dual diagnosis among older adults: cooccurring substance use disorders and psychiatric illness. *Journal of Dual Diagnosis* 2 (3): 9–30.

Blazer DG, Pennybacker MR (1984) Epidemiology of alcoholism in the elderly. In: Hartford JT, Samorajski T (eds). *Alcoholism in the Elderly.* New York: Raven Press, pp 25–33.

Blow FC, Cook CA, Booth BM, *et al.* (1991) Age-related psychiatric comorbidities and level of functioning in alcohol veterans seeking out-patient treatment. *Hospital and Community Psychiatry* 43: 990–995.

Brennan PL, Moos RH (1996) Late life drinking behaviour. *Alcohol Health & Research World* 20: 197–205.

Cabinet Office (2000) *Tackling Drugs to Build a Better Britain.* London: Central Office of Information.

Closser MH (1991) Benzodiazepine and the elderly. A review of potential problems. *Journal of Substance Abuse Treatment* 8 (1–2): 35–41.

Curtis J (1989) Characteristics, diagnosis and treatment of alcoholism in elderly patients. *Journal of American Geriatric Society* 37: 310–316.

Day E (2004) *Elderly risking health through binge drinking*. www.telegraph.co.uk.

Deblinger L (2000) Alcohol problems in the elderly. *Patient Care* 34: 70.

Department of Health (1995) *Sensible Drinking*. London: DH.

Department of Health (2002) *Mental Health Policy Implementation Guide: Dual Diagnosis Good Practice Guide*. London: Department of Health.

Department of Health (2005) *Everybody's Business*. London: DH.

Dunne FJ (1994) Misuse of drugs or drugs by elderly people. *British Medical Journal* 308 (6929): 608–609.

Ewing JA (1984) Detecting alcoholism – the CAGE questionnaire. *Journal of the American Medical Association* 252: 1905–1907.

Feuerlein W, Reiser E (1986) Parameters affecting the course and results of delirium tremens treatment. *Acta Psychiatrists Scandinavia Supplimentum* 329: 120–123.

Ghodse AH (1997) Substance misuse by the elderly. *British Journal of Hospital Medicine* 58 (9): 451–453.

Gilhooly M (2007) *Alcohol warning for older drinkers*. www.telegraph.co.uk.

Gulino C, Kadin M (1986) Aging Perspective of Alcoholism. *Geriatric Nursing* 7 (3): 148–151.

Hall C (2002) *Alcohol can help prevent dementia*. www.telegraph.co.uk

Hartford JT, Samorajski T (1982) Alcoholism in the geriatric population. *Journal of the Geriatric Society* 30: 18–24.

Highfield R (2008) *Drinking accelerates onset of Alzheimer's*. www.telegraph.co.uk.

Jones TV, Joseph C (1997) *Alcohol Use Disorders in the Older Adults: Clinical Guidelines*. New York: American Geriatric Society.

Kofoed LL (1985) OTC drug overdose in the elderly: what to watch for. *Geriatrics* 40 (10): 55–59.

Menninger JA (2002) Assessment and treatment of alcoholism and substance related disorders in the elderly. *Bulletin of the Menninger Clinic* 66: 166–184.

Miller WR, Rollnick S (1991) *Preparing People to Change Addictive Behaviour*. New York, London: The Guilford Press. p. 54.

Mishra B, Kastenbaum R (1980) Alcohol and old age. In: Ward M, Goodman C (eds). *Alcohol Problems in Old Age. A Practical Guide to Helping Older People with Alcohol Problems*. Wynne: Howard Publishing. pp 23–37.

Morgan K (1988) Hypnotic drug use for the elderly. *British Medical Journal* 296: 930.

Naik PC, Jones RG (1994) Alcohol histories taken from elderly people on admission. *British Medical Journal* 308 (6923): 248.

National Service Framework for Older People (2001) *Executive Summary*. London: Department of Health, HMSO.

Neve R (1993) Developments in drinking behaviour in the Netherlands. *Addiction* 88: 611–621.

Nutt D (2007) Development of a rationale scale to assess the harm of drugs of potential use. www.thelancet.com.

O'Connell H (2003) Alcohol use disorders in elderly people – re-defining an age old problem. *British Medical Journal* 327: 664–667.

Patterson TL, Jeste DV (1999) The potential impact of baby-boom generation on substance misuse among elderly persons. *Mental Health & Aging* 50 (9): 1184–1189.

Phillips P, Katz A (2001) Substance misuse in older adults: an emerging policy priority. *NT Research* 6: 898–905.

Reed J, Stanley C (2004) *Health Wellbeing and Older People*. Bristol: The Policy Press. pp 13–24.

Solfrizzi V, Panza F (2007) *Glass of wine a day 'fights off dementia'*. www.telegraph.co.uk

Swartz M, Landerman R, George LK (1991) Benzodiazepine anti anxiety agents: prevalence and correlates of use in southern community. *American Journal of Public Health* 81: 592–596.

Swift C (2001) Falls in later life and their consequences. *British Medical Journal* 322: 855–857.

Wright F, Whyley C (1994) *Accident Prevention and Risk Taking by Elderly People: The Need for Advice*. London: Age Concern Institute of Gerontology.

Chapter 11

Stimulant Use and Psychosis

Lorna Saunder

Introduction

Stimulant drugs include a wide range of substances, both legal and illegal. They exist on a continuum from the seemingly innocuous caffeine through the legal substances such as Khat and betel nut. The continuum then enters the illegal categories of substances such as the class B substance amphetamines (speed, whiz and billy), and finally the class A substances 3,4 methylenedioxy-N-methamphetamine (MDMA) (ecstasy and its derivative 3,4 methylenedioxyamphetamine (MDA)) and cocaine (charlie and coke), also known in its smokable form as crack (rocks, white and stones).

The vast majority of people in the United Kingdom use stimulants such as cups of tea and coffee, cans of cola drinks, energy drinks and chocolate, whether they are aware of it or not. All of these everyday substances have a powerful impact upon our perceived energy levels and functioning. Yet more powerful stimulants can have a devastating effect on the body and mind. Sustained use of stimulants such as cocaine and amphetamine can push the body beyond its natural capability. The body's basic restorative functions such as eating and sleeping can be impaired to a dangerous degree. In addition, the toxic effects of these substances include cardiac damage, fits, strokes and malnutrition to name but a few. If these effects are observed physiologically, then what effect can be observed on the mind?

The aim of this chapter is to look more closely at the effects of the three most widely used illegal stimulant drugs, amphetamines, ecstasy and cocaine, particularly in relation to psychotic illness. Where information is available regarding specific substances, then this will be named. Where the term stimulant is used, the reader should assume that the author is referring to the common effects that all of these substances have, i.e. sleeplessness, suppressed appetite, tachycardia and increased levels of dopamine and serotonin in the brain.

Stimulant use in the United Kingdom

The British Crime Survey 2003/2004 (Chivite Matthews *et al.* 2005) revealed that drug use is highest in England and Wales. It showed that of adults aged 16–59, 35.6% had tried an illegal drug at some point in their lives. In terms of specific substances, the use rates break down as follows.

British Crime Survey 2003/2004

Lifetime prevalence rates of those aged 16–59:

Cannabis	30.8%
Amphetamines	12.2%
Hallucinogens	9.4%
Ecstasy	6.9%
Cocaine	6.2%
Crack	0.2%
Opiates	0.8%

If the results are broken down, the *British Crime Survey 2003/2004* shows that for the 16–24 age group, the use of any drug has decreased and the use of class A drugs has remained stable since 1998. If the 16–59 age group is looked at as a whole, overall drug use has remained stable but class A drug use has increased, with a particular increase in cocaine use. To put these statistics into context, it means that around 11 million people in the United Kingdom aged 16–59 have used illicit drugs at some point in their lives; of these around 4 million have used a class A drug in their lifetime. In comparison, a large and significant study by Menezes *et al.* (1996) looked at a sample of 171 people suffering from psychotic illnesses and they revealed a lifetime prevalence rate of amphetamines of 12.9%. This is slightly higher than the general population. This study is of key importance because it is one of the largest and most rigorous of its kind undertaken within the United Kingdom. Margolese *et al.* (2004) examined substance use among people diagnosed with schizophrenia and psychotic illnesses in Canada. They found very low rates of stimulant use. A lifetime rate of cocaine use of 3.9% of the sample was reported. The authors compared this to the United States where lifetime rates among this population are reported to be as high as 10–15%.

Stimulants and drug-induced psychosis

There has been a significant amount of debate regarding the term drug-induced psychosis with many people believing it is an umbrella term. It is

widely used for people experiencing psychotic symptoms following ingestion of substances. Strang and Farrell (1994) break this down into two separate
categories. These are drug-induced disorders and drug-precipitated disorders. A drug-induced psychosis occurs often as a result of ingestion of a large
amount of stimulant (Curran *et al*. 2004) and is primarily a toxic response.
When considering the relationship between stimulant use, drug-induced
psychosis and the development of longer tem mental health problems, Hambrecht and Häfner (2003) support the argument that a true drug-induced
psychosis should only last for the duration of the drug effects, and the
following quote illustrates this further.

> *Psychotic states beyond a duration of three weeks after cessation of drug intake
> should not be considered to be only a drug-induced psychosis.* Hambrecht and
> Häfner (2003)

Cocaine and amphetamine have been particularly associated with these
kinds of responses (Strang *et al*. 1993; Withers *et al*. 1995; Srisurapanont *et al*.
2001). In an extensive review of research, Murray (1998) reports on studies
whereby individuals have been given high doses of amphetamines and psychotic illnesses resembling paranoid schizophrenia have emerged. Strang
et al. (1993) describes psychosis induced by cocaine as being short-lived at
around 24 hours, depending on the dosage. The psychosis will resolve when
the body has been able to metabolise the offending substance. Strang *et al*.
(1993) also discuss cocaine hallucinosis in which the user experiences some
hallucinations, may be paranoid and will have impaired insight although
insight is not absent altogether. This may lead to cocaine psychosis, which
may be characterised by persecutory delusions and more vivid hallucinations. This is supported by Cubells *et al*. (2005) who found that groups of
people experiencing cocaine-induced psychosis primarily experienced auditory and visual hallucinations, persecutory delusions and paranoia. Vaiva
et al. (2001) drew conclusions from a case study whereby a psychotic disorder was precipitated by MDMA (ecstasy). In this study, the psychotic illness
lasted longer than would be expected from a toxic drug-induced psychosis.
Cassidy and Ballard (1994) also supported this through two case study
reports. It would appear that a psychotic illness could be precipitated but
does not necessarily progress to long-term psychotic illness. This finding was
supported by an individual case study by Series *et al*. (1994). The difference
in this case was that the individual had no preceding mental health problem
and had used ecstasy in isolation. The use of other substances often clouds
the clinical picture and ecstasy is frequently accompanied by the use of
other stimulants and cannabis, all of which are associated with psychotic
reactions (Maxwell 2003). Case studies are useful in terms of sharing clinical experience but provide little in the way of valid argument as they are

unsupported by rigorous research and these case studies are quite old. Lieb *et al.* (2002) and Parrott and Turner (2000) also reported poly substance use among ecstasy users and these were much more methodologically sound studies. Parrott *et al.* (2000) compared a group of 12 heavy ecstasy users, 16 light ecstasy users and 22 non-ecstasy users. This study is useful to consider because despite the small numbers the participants were recruited via the snowball method within a local community. The significance of the snowball method is that it is a way of contacting people who are using substances but are not presenting to services with problem drug use. This means that the participants may be less likely to be suffering from any of the vulnerabilities to addiction and mental illness that requires professional help. Of the group, the heavy ecstasy users reported the highest scores for a range of mental health problems including psychosis. The group of light ecstasy users reported higher scores than the non-users on only two areas, which were psychoticism and paranoid ideation. The conclusions from this study were that heavy ecstasy use certainly increased the risk for psychological problems but that even light use could affect a person's mental health. The authors of this study recognised strongly that these findings must be treated with caution as all of the participants were using other substances. The authors recognise the difficulty of finding people who use ecstasy in isolation without concurrent use of cannabis, cocaine and hallucinogens. Until robust studies with people who use ecstasy in isolation are undertaken on a large scale, it will be extremely difficult to truly determine its effect on mental health and its relationship with psychotic illness. Landabaso *et al.* (2002) undertook a study with 32 people who had presented with ecstasy-related psychosis. The initial sample was larger, but the researchers excluded anyone with a prior history of psychosis (23.2% of the original sample) and people using substances other than ecstasy. Of the sample, the symptoms that were observed most frequently were the so-called positive symptoms such as hallucinations, although there were also negative symptoms (blunted affect and depression) present. In terms of the progression of illness, the majority of the subjects experienced severe symptoms in the first month. Symptoms were moderate by 3 months, with a significant reduction in depressive symptoms and by 6 months, the symptoms were no longer clinically relevant. The participants in this study were treated with olanzapine during this time. Some caution must be exercised when considering these findings because as the authors point out, there was no control group used to compare with; therefore, there is no way of proving whether this improvement in symptoms would have occurred naturally or were a response to medical intervention. However, what is really remarkable about this study is that there was a retention rate of 96.9% of those who completed the 6-month program. This level of completion is extremely unusual and the authors fail to give any reasons for this. There could, therefore, be a question over the participants in the study being more motivated than normal, which may have influenced the progress of their illness. Creighton *et al.* (1991) likens the psychotic states induced by ecstasy to that of LSD. This is because although ecstasy is classed as a stimulant, it has a much more hallucinogenic effect than cocaine or amphetamine. However, Creighton *et al.* (1991) also go onto say that it must be remembered that given the number of people who report using ecstasy the numbers reporting adverse effects are actually very low.

The scope of this chapter does not allow for a full examination of other stimulant substances such as Khat and there is also a paucity of research in this area. However, Cox and Rampes (2003) report incidents of Khat causing short-lived schizophreniform illness and that this toxic response is less frequent than that caused by amphetamine. As reported by other authors, this response is seen to be dose dependent and resolves within 3–4 days. The difficulty in looking at research relating to Khat is that many Khat users are immigrants and often do not contact services. This makes accurate detection of the incidence of Khat-related illness difficult.

Another issue to consider when trying to determine the effects of stimulant use is sensitisation to substances, which also ties in with Strang and Farrell's (1994) consideration of drug-precipitated disorder. Williams and Farrell (2004) suggest that repeated psychotic episodes of stimulant use result in the individuals' psychotic threshold being lowered, and lower doses of the substance can trigger a psychotic episode. Hence, instead of drawing the conclusion that stimulants cause long-term mental health problems, it could also be posited that an individual may become more susceptible over time to the effects of stimulants and the illness is characterised by repeated episodes. A study that supports this theory of sensitisation is by Yui *et al.* (2001). In this study a group of female Japanese prisoners who had previously experienced methamphetamine-induced psychosis were examined for evidence of recurrent psychotic episodes, which the authors term *flashbacks*. This study's strengths come from the inclusion of a control group, that the participants did not use any other substances during the study (owing to the Japanese penal system's strict control of substances) and that the participants had had no previous mental health problems in the absence of methamphetamine use. Of the group of women who had experienced methamphetamine psychosis, 50% of them had reoccurrences during their incarceration. When examined more closely, these occurrences occurred when the women were exposed to mild psychosocial stressors. These stressors were also experienced by the control group but did not result in a psychotic reaction. Within the group was a sub-group that experienced persistent psychotic reactions to methamphetamine use and all of these women had had frightening experiences while using methamphetamine. The authors of this study also examined closely the biological responses in this group of women and found that those with noradrenergic hyperactivity and increased dopamine levels were most likely to experience recurrent psychotic episodes. This study adds a strong argument to support the idea of sensitisation in the brains of people who experience psychotic reactions following stimulant use. However, it was a reasonably small study with 80 participants, of whom 39 had methamphetamine psychosis. The fact that it was undertaken in Japan may also make its findings difficult to apply in the United Kingdom, mainly because we have little methamphetamine use in the United Kingdom although it is on the rise. In addition, the participants were inmates in prison and it could be argued that when the association with criminal behaviour and mental illness is considered, this group of women may have been more likely to develop mental illness anyway. A larger study by Cubells *et al.* (2005) examined the experiences of 181 people suffering from cocaine-induced paranoia. Of this group, 84% denied experiencing paranoia upon their first use of cocaine and 72.2% then stated that using greater amounts of cocaine increased the paranoia. The authors argue that this adds support to the sensitisation argument. This is because the paranoia symptoms worsen over time and with greater expo-sure to the substance, although without thorough laboratory testing, this is likely to be difficult to prove, but this study does include a good-sized sample of subjects.

The picture is rarely clear when considering the effects of substance use upon an individual's mental health and it is commonly accepted that indi-viduals suffering from a drug-induced psychotic illness will tend to exhibit more florid psychotic symptoms, which is how it is differentiated from a schizophrenia-type illness that will have negative symptoms such as anhe-donia and thought disturbance. A small study by Harris and Batki (2000) disproved this as their participants who had stimulant-induced psychosis were clearly exhibiting negative symptamology. This finding must be con-sidered carefully as one of the clear flaws of the study was that there was no differentiation between the participants as to whether they were in acute intoxication or withdrawal states, which is likely to cloud the clinical picture significantly.

Stimulants and mental illness

As with all areas of dual diagnosis study, there is always the chicken and egg argument with regard to whether the metal illness or substance use comes first, which makes the causal relationship unclear. In a report by Schifano (2001), 150 poly drug users who have used ecstasy were asked about their mental health problems. Fifty-three per cent reported one or more disorders, which were mainly depression and psychosis. There is no mention of whether these illnesses preceded the drug use, and the users were not using ecstasy in isolation. In a review of 127 articles relating to treatment of co-occurring mental illness and substance use, Watkins *et al.* (2005) came to the following conclusion:

> *Although mental disorders may be the result of substance abuse, epidemiologic data indicate that most mental disorders temporally precede substance abuse, which suggests that they are two independent disorders and that the substance use is exacerbating rather than causing the mental disorder.* Watkins *et al.* (2005)

This finding was also supported by an extensive longitudinal study by Lieb *et al.* (2002). A total of 3021 German people were interviewed, of which 8.9% reported having used ecstasy. From this sample 68.7% of them reported a history of DSM IV disorders (substance use disorders, affective disorders, anxiety disorders, somatoform and eating disorders). Of this group that had experienced mental disorder, the vast majority (88.4%) had a clearly occurring mental disorder that preceded the ecstasy use. Given the size of this study and the fact that it is longitudinal, the results are significant in terms of consideration given to ecstasy as a causative factor in the development of mental illness. This study shows that a small number of people do develop mental health difficulties following ecstasy use but for the vast majority they were already experiencing mental health problems. Unfortunately, this study looks into neither the relationship between ecstasy and psychosis nor at the effect ecstasy has had on people with existing psychotic illnesses. In addition, it must be borne in mind that it was undertaken in Germany, which may have a different mental health profile to that in the United Kingdom. The prevalence of ecstasy use within the population studied was higher than that found in the United Kingdom.

Stimulants and their use by people with existing psychotic illnesses

An extensive review of literature by Curran *et al.* (2004) revealed that a single dose of stimulants could increase psychosis ratings in 50–70% of the participants who had schizophrenia or acute psychotic symptoms. Curran *et al.* (2004) also went on to say that compliance with medication will not prevent a relapse or worsening of symptoms when stimulants are used. It is often assumed when people who use stimulants and have a psychotic illness have a relapse that they have been non-compliant with medication, which can lead to mistrust within the therapeutic alliance. The review by Srisurapanont *et al.* (2001) identifies antipsychotics having a positive effect on people experiencing psychosis following the use of amphetamines. It could therefore be argued that people with an existing psychotic illness when exposed to stimulants have an altered response. If the individual without a psychotic illness responds well to antipsychotics after exposure to stimulants and makes little difference for the person with a psychotic illness, then there could be an argument made for sensitisation. Sensitisation would suggest that individuals with pre-existing psychotic illnesses are somehow more sensitive to the psychoactive effects of stimulants, although there is little data to support this currently. This sensitisation may account for a finding by Dixon (1999) in which people with a secondary psychotic illness were more likely than people with schizophrenia to use cocaine. If people with schizophrenia are sensitised to the effects of cocaine, then a heightened response may be unpleasant. It could also be argued that people with schizophrenia are less likely to use cocaine for social reasons such as lack of money, social skills, etc.

In a fascinating study by Lahti *et al.* (2001), they compared the effect of ketamine on people with and without schizophrenia. Although ketamine is not strictly a stimulant drug, it is a drug that is commonly used alongside stimulants within the club scene in the United Kingdom. This study was undertaken in order to find a drug that mimics schizophrenic symptoms in unaffected volunteers so that pharmacological research can be undertaken. The outcome of this study was that the people with schizophrenia showed no increase in their negative symptoms and their positive symptoms increased but to the same degree as the unaffected volunteers. The relevance of this study to this discussion is that there is often an assumption that certain substances have a catastrophic effect on people with schizophrenia, but this study showed that the administration of a substance to this group showed no worse deterioration than in the unaffected volunteers, and their baseline mental health status returned to normal very quickly. Without further studies like this, it is difficult to draw accurate conclusions about the effect of stimulant use on people with schizophrenia; however, the ethical issues regarding the testing of psychoactive substances on people with an existing severe mental health problem would preclude this.

In terms of the response of people with schizophrenia to substances, a relatively rigorous study by Margolese *et al.* (2004) clearly revealed that substance abuse affects the positive but not the negative symptoms of schizophrenia. Although as with many studies of this kind, it relies on self-report data that can be viewed as unreliable, particularly in people who may have some cognitive deterioration as a result of their mental health problems or from treatment with psychoactive medication. However, it is useful for clinicians to bear in mind these findings when considering a service user's illness progression. Deterioration in someone's negative symptoms may be attributed to substance use and be incorrectly treated.

CASE STUDY 1

Robbie is a 22-year-old Caucasian man, who is suffering from a psychotic illness that has resulted in admission to acute psychiatric services on a number of occasions. All of Robbie's admissions have been preceded by episodes of stimulant use. However, he is beginning to show some worrying symptoms such as social withdrawal and anhedonia; at this stage schizophrenia is suspected.

Robbie's first contact with mental health services occurred at age 19. He had been studying for his 'A' levels but had dropped out of the program. His parents had become increasingly worried about Robbie's behaviour. At this stage they were unaware of Robbie's drug taking. Robbie had become increasingly paranoid and, at times, appeared to be suffering from persecutory delusions. This culminated in Robbie arriving at the family home one night extremely agitated and with pressure of speech. He was convinced his parents had been watching him through closed-circuit television (CCTV) in the house and he smashed the house up in an attempt to locate the cameras. The police were called and Robbie was eventually detained under section 2.

Following his first admission, a urine drug screen was undertaken and Robbie tested positive for cocaine and cannabis. He denied using any drugs and was reluctant to discuss any of his symptoms. He was given a low dose of antipsychotics, which he responded to well. Robbie was discharged with minimal follow-up and his illness was labelled a drug-induced psychosis.

Within 3 months Robbie was admitted again under similar circumstances. This time he was detained under section 3 of the Mental Health Act (MHA). Robbie formed a positive relationship with a dual diagnosis nurse who visited Robbie from the community mental health team. Robbie was able to admit that he had begun using amphetamines at age 14; he then began using ecstasy at 16. At this stage he was using these substances irregularly. At age 18 he began using cocaine with his friends; this was initially occasional use. By age 19 he wanted to use cocaine on a near daily basis; however, his finances would not allow it. So he interspersed his cocaine use with amphetamines. Eventually, he began smoking cocaine as crack and was using high levels of alcohol and cannabis to come down.

Robbie was again discharged but this time given antipsychotics and follow-up with the dual diagnosis nurse. He maintained this regime for a few months and even considered returning to college. He then ceased contact with services. The breakdown of a relationship triggered another binge, which ended up in an admission via accident and emergency after Robbie had been found unconscious. When he regained consciousness he was responding to voices and appeared to be actively hallucinating. Robbie's recovery took much longer this time and he frequently complained that none of his friends wanted to know him any more. He had become more withdrawn and anhedonic and he spent long periods sleeping and had begun to neglect his self-care. Robbie was eventually discharged after 5 months. He remains in contact with a dual diagnosis nurse in the community and remains on medication. He has had episodes of use but there have been no binges. This episodic use is usually triggered by meeting with certain friends. Robbie's consultant is currently considering a diagnosis of schizophrenia.

Implications for practice

A key element in caring for people with substance misuse and mental health issues is the therapeutic alliance formed between service user and carer. A review of substance misuse literature by Meier *et al.* (2005) revealed a key finding that an early therapeutic alliance was 'a constant predictor of engagement and retention in drug treatment'. This review of the literature only took into account service users who had substance misuse issues rather than a dual diagnosis. An interesting study by Petry and Bickel (1999) examined the added factor of psychopathology when considering the effect of the therapeutic alliance with opiate users. One hundred and fourteen people in a treatment program were rated on their therapeutic alliance with their therapists. This was undertaken from the therapist's point of view and that of the patients. One of the key findings was that the therapeutic alliance was a key factor in the treatment outcome. Twenty-three per cent of the patients with moderate-to-severe psychiatric symptoms and below average therapeutic alliance scores completed treatment compared with 75% of people with the same degree of psychiatric symptoms but were scoring highly on the therapeutic alliance scores. This study would indicate that treatment outcomes could be improved threefold by the presence of a positive therapeutic alliance. The study is limited because although there were a large number of participants, only three therapists were used. This could indicate some degree of bias in that the therapeutic alliances formed were peculiar to those therapists and this relationship was not examined in detail. Barber *et al.* (1999) used ratings scales of therapeutic alliance with 252 people receiving outpatient treatment for cocaine dependence found that therapeutic alliance had little impact upon subjects completing the therapeutic program. This group did suffer from a high dropout rate and the people who dropped out were subsequently included in the study, which may have influenced the results. At the end of the study, the authors did discover that early treatment alliance resulted in a longer time spent in treatment, although they do state that this finding would require further testing as it was not an initial research question. Carey (1996) recommends specific strategies in building a therapeutic alliance as 'providing medications, assistance in obtaining entitlements, food and recreational opportunities'. When working with service users such as Robbie it is also vital that practitioners have an understanding of the service users' reality, especially in terms of their drug use. It is all very well enticing people into treatment with the promise of sorting out benefits and recreational opportunities, but it is also vital that the staff working with service users such as Robbie have a thorough understanding of substance use. This knowledge should be current and focused on routes of administration, costs and effects. McLaughlin *et al.* (2000) outlined this in a small study undertaken with drug users in Northern Ireland. One of the key findings of this study was that drug users perceived many healthcare workers to be lacking in knowledge and skills related to the care of drug users. This group of people felt that when healthcare workers had a credible level of knowledge they responded more positively to them.

In working with Robbie it is important to understand the reasons for his continued substance use in the face of experiencing such negative outcomes. In a comparative study of people with major affective disorder and schizophrenia, Gearon *et al.* (2001) interviewed 25 people with schizophrenia regarding their motivations for drug use. A key finding was that people with schizophrenia were more likely than those with major affective disorder to report drug us as a response to social and environmental factors. The participants also did not report use as a way of self-medicating unpleasant symptoms but did use as a result of peer pressure and boredom. In this study cocaine use was reported more widely than cannabis use, which may be accounted for by the different patterns of drug use in the United States. It should be borne in mind that people use different drugs for different reasons and if it had solely focused on stimulant use, the outcome may have been different. The authors also identified that the data collected were via self-report. Self-report in substance misuse research is often criticised for its lack of accuracy and may be seen as a methodological weakness. If we apply the findings of this study to Robbie's case, it could be suggested that a focus of treatment could be to consider his social and environmental stressors such as peer pressure and boredom. This suggestion would be supported by reference to the literature review undertaken by Meier *et al.* (2005), whereby a strong social network was also a key indicator in the recovery from substance misuse.

In terms of pharmacological treatment, it has already been suggested that olanzapine has a good effect on stimulant-related psychotic symptoms (Landabaso *et al.* 2002). If Robbie's condition deteriorated any further and clozapine was considered, it may be worth considering the following study by Farren *et al.* (2000). In this study non-psychotic subjects were pre-treated with ascending doses of clozapine (up to 50 mg). They were then given pharmaceutical doses of cocaine. It was found that the clozapine reduced the high felt by the users following the administration of cocaine. This finding may be important in reducing the reinforcing effect of cocaine use. However, the study was extremely small with only eight subjects and authors urging caution in prescribing clozapine to known cocaine users owing to an increased cocaine serum level following clozapine administration and also the potential cardiac complications known with both drugs. This study only reports on the physiological effects of the combination of clozapine and cocaine and does not consider the psychological effects to any great degree.

When working with Robbie his community dual diagnosis nurse opted to loosely follow the program outlined by Bellack and Gearon (1998). This is because it is a program of interventions that was developed with a group of patients who were suffering from schizophrenia and their primary substance of use was cocaine. The philosophy of this program is to use a lot of behavioural rehearsal and use of handouts and memory prompts in order to counteract the cognitive deficits that occur as a result of the schizophrenia. The key areas that were focused on in Robbie's treatment are as follows:

- Social skills training – developing non-substance using contacts, refusal skills;
- Education – effects of substances, triggers for use, craving, effect on mental health;
- Goal setting;
- Behavioural skills – coping with high-risk situations and relapse prevention.

Conclusion

The conclusions that can be drawn from this chapter should be considered by all practitioners working with clients who are suffering from psychotic symptoms and use stimulant drugs. It should be considered that, in the same way, stimulant drugs exist on a continuum and so do psychotic illnesses. These illnesses range from the toxic response of a drug-induced psychosis, which should resolve quickly and leave the person unharmed. Then comes a more severe drug-precipitated psychosis, which may have longer term consequences, although what we primarily see in these cases is that the individuals concerned frequently have a mental illness preceding the substance use. Finally, we see people with schizophrenia who use stimulant substances and see a worsening of positive symptoms. In terms of clinical practice, the research reviewed in this chapter supports the argument towards some kind of sensitisation process following a psychotic response to stimulants. Clinicians should ensure that this information is given to people suffering drug-induced or drug-precipitated psychotic episodes in order to prevent recurrence. Clinicians should also not underestimate the significance of the therapeutic alliance and should tailor interventions according to the capabilities of the service user. Finally, credibility and knowledge are vital in the care and treatment of this group of people.

References

Barber J, Luborsky L, Crits-Christoph P, *et al.* (1999) Therapeutic alliance as a predictor of outcome in treatment of cocaine dependence. *Psychotherapy Research* 9 (1): 54–73.

Bellack A, Gearon J (1998) Substance abuse treatment for people with schizophrenia. *Addictive Behaviors* 23 (6): 749–766.

Carey K (1996) Substance use reduction in the context of outpatient psychiatric treatment: a collaborative, motivational harm reduction approach. *Community Mental Health Journal* 32 (3): 291–306.

Cassidy G, Ballard C (1994) Psychiatric sequelae of MDMA (ecstasy) and related drugs. *Irish Journal of Psychological Medicine* 11 (3): 132–133.

Chivite Matthews N, Richardson A, O'Shea J, *et al*. (2005) *Drug Misuse Declared: Findings from the British Crime Survey 2003/2004. Home Office Statistical Bulletin*. Available: http://www.homeoffice.gov.uk/rds/pdfs05/hosb0405.pdf (1.11.2005).

Cox G, Rampes H (2003) Adverse effects of Khat: a review. *Advances in Psychiatric Treatment* 9: 456–463.

Creighton FJ, Black DL, Hyde CE (1991) "Ecstasy" psychosis and flashbacks. *British Journal of Psychiatry* 159: 713–715.

Cubells J, Feinn R, Pearson D, *et al*. (2005) Rating the severity and character of transient cocaine-induced delusions and hallucinations with a new instrument, the Scale for Assessment of Positive Symptoms for Cocaine Induced Psychosis (SAPS-CIP). *Drug and Alcohol Dependence* 80 (1): 23–33.

Curran C, Byrappa N, McBride A (2004) Stimulant psychosis: systematic review. *The British Journal of Psychiatry* 185: 196–204.

Dixon L (1999) Dual diagnosis substance abuse in schizophrenia: prevalence and impact on outcomes. *Schizophrenia Research* 35: 93–100.

Farren C, Hameedi F, Rosen M, *et al*. (2000) Significant interaction between clozapine and cocaine in cocaine addicts. *Drug and Alcohol Dependence* 59 (2): 153–163.

Gearon J, Bellack A, Rachbeisel J, Dixon L (2001) Drug use behaviour and correlates in people with schizophrenia. *Addictive Behaviors* 26: 51–61.

Hambrecht M, Häfner H (2003) Temporal order and aetiology. In: Graham H, Copello A, Birchwood M, Mueser K (eds). *Substance Misuse in Psychosis: Approaches to Treatment and Service Delivery*, 1st Edition. Chichester: John Wiley and Sons.

Harris D, Batki S (2000) Stimulant psychosis: symptom profile and acute clinical course. *The American Journal of Addictions* 9: 28–37.

Lahti A, Weiler M, Michaelidis T, Parwani A, Tamminga C (2001) Effects of ketamine in normal and schizophrenic volunteers. *Neuropyschobiopharmacology* 25 (4): 455–467.

Landabaso M, Iraurgi I, Jimenez-Lerma J, *et al*. (2002) Ecstasy-induced psychotic disorder: six month follow up study. *European Addiction Research* 8 (3): 133–140.

Lieb R, Schuetz C, Pfister H, von Sydow K, Wittchen U (2002) Mental disorders in ecstasy users: a prospective longitudinal investigation. *Drug and Alcohol Dependence* 68 (2): 195–207.

Margolese H, Malchy L, Negrete J, Tempier R, Gill K (2004) Drug and alcohol use among patients with schizophrenia and related psychoses: levels and consequences. *Schizophrenia Research* 67 (2–3): 157–166.

Maxwell J (2003) Response to club drug use. *Current Opinion in Psychiatry* 16 (3): 279–289.

McLaughlin D, McKenna H, Leslie J (2000) The perceptions and aspirations illicit drug users hold toward health care staff and the care they receive. *Journal of Psychiatric and Mental Health Nursing* 7: 435–441.

Meier P, Barrowclough C, Donmall M (2005) The role of the therapeutic alliance in the treatment of substance misuse: a critical review of the literature. *Addiction* 100 (3): 304–316.

Menezes P, Johnson S, Thornicroft G, *et al.* (1996) Drug and alcohol problems among individuals with severe mental illness in south London. *British Journal of Psychiatry* 168 (5): 612–619.

Murray J (1998) Psychophysiological aspects of amphetamine and methamphetamine abuse. *Journal of Psychology* 132 (2): 227–237.

Parrott AC, Sisk E, Turner J (2000) Psychobiological problems in heavy "ecstasy" (MDMA) polydrug users. *Drug and Alcohol Dependence* 60 (1): 105–110.

Petry N, Bickel W (1999) Therapeutic alliance and psychiatric severity as predictors of completion of treatment for opioid dependence. *Psychiatric Services* (50): 219–227.

Schifano F (2001) Long term effects of ecstasy consumption. *Substance Misuse Bulletin* 14 (1): 6–7.

Series H, Boeles S, Dorkins E, Peveler R (1994) Psychiatric complications of "ecstasy" use. *Journal of Psychopharmacology* 8 (1): 60–61.

Srisurapanont M, Kittiratanapaiboon P, Jarasuraisin N (2001) Treatment for amphetamine psychosis. *The Cochrane Database of Systematic Reviews* (4), Art no: CD003026. DOI: 10. 1002/14651858. CD003026.

Strang J, Farrell M (1994) Illicit drug use: clinical features and treatment. In: Chick J, Cantwell R (eds). *Seminars in Alcohol and Drug Misuse*. London: Gaskell, p. 38.

Strang J, Johns A, Caan W (1993) Cocaine in the UK 1991. *British Journal of Psychiatry* 162: 1–13.

Vaiva G, Boss V, Bailly D, *et al.* (2001) An "accidental" acute psychosis with ecstasy use. *Journal of Psychoactive Drugs* 33 (1): 95–97.

Watkins K, Hunter S, Burnham A, Pincus H, Nicholson G (2005) Review of treatment for person with co-occurring affective or anxiety and substance use disorder. *Psychiatric Services* 56 (8): 913–926

Williams A, Farrell M (2004) Substance use and psychosis. *Psychiatry* 3 (1): 52–54.

Withers N, Pulvirenti L, Koob G, Gillin C (1995) Cocaine abuse and dependence. *Journal of Clinical Psychopharmacology* 15 (1): 63–77.

Yui K, Goto K, Ikemoto S, *et al.* (2001) Susceptibility to subsequent episodes of spontaneous recurrence of methamphetamine psychosis. *Drug and Alcohol Dependence* 64 (2): 133–142.

Chapter 12

Women and Dual Diagnosis

Julie Winnington

Introduction

The incidence of a dual diagnosis in substance misusers is similar in both genders; however, there is a marked difference in the types of mental health diagnoses in men and women. Women with a substance misuse problem are more likely to suffer from affective disorder, whereas men are more likely to have a diagnosis of schizophrenia or personality disorder, particularly antisocial personality disorder.

Women tend to be more reluctant to disclose substance misuse and are more likely to present to their general practitioner (GP) or mental health services with symptoms of mental illness compared to men who are more likely to present directly to addiction services (Turning Point & Rethink 2004). Consequently, the substance misuse problem is picked up much later in their drug-using career or may be missed altogether, sometimes leading to a misdiagnosis.

Women who misuse substances are significantly more likely than other women or men to have experienced sexual, physical and/or emotional abuse as children (Galvani and Humphreys 2007) and are, therefore, more likely to show symptoms of post-traumatic stress disorder (PTSD). The cycle of abuse may be perpetuated in adulthood, with women more likely than men to have a drug-using partner, and substance misuse lifestyles often include sex working for women, an occupation that carries a high risk of sexual assault.

It is estimated that two-thirds of all drug users are men, with these figures replicated in those seeking substance specific treatment. Very few Tier 2 and 3 gender-specific services exist, which may provide a barrier for women entering or remaining in treatment. Mixed gender residential facilities for detoxification and/or rehabilitation may also prevent women seeking treatment or may have an adverse impact on their ability to engage with therapeutic programmes.

Although this chapter focuses on co-occurring mental health problems and substance misuse, it is important to make reference to the poor physical health of women with a dual diagnosis. Women substance misusers suffer from physical complications at an earlier stage, and at a lower rate of use than males (Califano 2006). In drug-using populations, women have higher rates of HIV than men and tend to inject earlier in their drug-using careers than men.

It has been suggested that women need more support for a longer time than men in order to achieve abstinence and good mental health (Messina *et al.* 2000), which should be taken into account by service providers.

Gender differences in dual diagnosis

Men with a dual diagnosis are more likely to have a diagnosis of schizophrenia, whereas women are more likely to suffer from an affective disorder. Many studies have examined the correlation of childhood sexual abuse and subsequent substance misuse. It is estimated that as many as 50–90% of women abusing substances suffered childhood sexual abuse, with the figures for men estimated between 20 and 40%, rates considerably higher than in the general population.

Women are more susceptible than men to substance misuse-related interpersonal problems, trauma and medical problems (Greenfield *et al.* 2003). One of the reasons for this may be that women who abuse substances often have substance-misusing partners who may continue the pattern of abuse. Women are more likely to share injecting equipment with a sexual partner than men, leading to increased rates of HIV among female IV drug users. Women are also more prone to physical complications as a result of their drug and alcohol use than men.

Personality disorders are also more prevalent in a substance-misusing population. Women are more likely to be diagnosed with a borderline personality disorder, with a ratio of 7:3. Seventy percent of those diagnosed had experienced childhood sexual abuse. Borderline personality disorder symptoms include feeling 'empty', anxious or depressed, impulsivity, self-harm and a difficulty in controlling emotions. In men with a substance misuse problem, antisocial or dis-social personality disorder is the most prevalent. This is characterised by not caring about the feelings of others, tendency towards aggression and criminal behaviour, being easily frustrated, impulsivity and the apparent inability to learn from unpleasant experiences.

PTSD, particularly complex PTSD, can be easily misdiagnosed as borderline personality disorder. The rates of childhood sexual abuse among attenders of drug treatment services are very high, with studies citing between 50 and 90% of women and between 20 and 42% of men; thus, it is likely that many will show symptoms of complex PTSD. Complex PTSD often occurs in those who suffered a trauma in childhood, and where the trauma goes on for a long time, rather than being an isolated event, and is caused by a parent or care giver. PTSD symptoms include flashbacks and nightmares, numbing, avoidance and hypervigilance. These symptoms are often relieved by the use of substances. In complex PTSD additional symptoms such as physical symptoms, self-harm and suicide and risk taking behaviours also occur. As substance misuse can mask many of these symptoms and also work as a memory suppressor, there may be a resurgence of these symptoms during detoxification. If these symptoms become unbearable during detoxification, it is likely that the client will drop out of treatment; thus, skilled interventions are required to support the client during this time.

CASE STUDY 1

Kathy, a 34-year-old, was referred to her local community drug services. She had been attending her GP surgery frequently over the last few years, with intermittent, severe stomach pains with no apparent physical cause. She also complained of depressive symptoms, such as low mood and sleep problems. Prescribed medication did not relieve the pain, so after being introduced through a friend, she began to use heroin. At the time she engaged with drug services, she was injecting heroin around three times daily and had also begun to take illicit benzodiazepines to aid sleep. It emerged during the course of her treatment with the drug services that she had suffered severe, prolonged sexual abuse as a child, and her stomach pains could be dated from that time. She was referred to her local psychology team where she received treatment for complex PTSD. Her stomach pains gradually receded, her mood lifted and she was able to begin reducing her drug use.

Eating disorders occur marginally more frequently in women than in men, and in those with a diagnosis of eating disorder there is a higher rate of reported substance misuse than in the general population. Female alcoholics, perhaps unsurprisingly considering the high calorific value of alcoholic drinks, are far less likely than the general population to suffer from anorexia, but have a higher incidence of bulimia, characterised by binge eating and induced vomiting. These figures reverse in the case of problematic drug users, with anorexia being particularly associated with crack and heroin use, crack cocaine having the useful effect of appetite suppression.

Depressive symptoms are common in all of those seeking treatment for substance misuse. In women, these symptoms are more likely to pre-date their substance misuse (Moscato et al. 1998), whereas depression in men is more likely to be an effect of the substance misuse. In both genders depressive symptoms tend to improve within the first 1–3 months of abstinence or substitute prescribing. Therefore, close monitoring of mood during the early stages of drug treatment will enable an accurate diagnosis and reduce unnecessary prescribing of antidepressants. Most alcoholics will report periods of extreme sadness during their drinking careers, but few will require pharmacological intervention once abstinence has been achieved.

Both women and men with a diagnosis of schizophrenia and substance misuse are more likely to come into contact with mental health rather than drug services.

A risk for both genders is a false diagnosis of schizophrenia due to self-reporting of schizophrenic symptoms, which were caused either by intoxication or withdrawal. This will be especially true for women who, as discussed earlier, are less likely to disclose substance misuse.

CASE STUDY 2

Grace, who is in her mid-forties, was first diagnosed with schizophrenia when she was a teenager. She suffered many negative effects as a result of her illness, including anhedonia and lethargy, and found it difficult socialising with others. She had tried many different illicit drugs since her teens. Her current drug of choice was amphetamine sulphate, which she found eased the negative symptoms of her schizophrenia and she stated that when she used amphetamines she had more energy and was more able to cope with the demands of daily life. Grace was receiving medication for her schizophrenia from her GP and buying amphetamines illicitly. She was then referred to her local dual diagnosis service, who, over a long period of time, found a prescribed medication that suited her and helped alleviate many of her symptoms, as well as did relapse prevention work with her. Over this period Grace was able to reduce and then eventually stop her amphetamine use.

The impact of dual diagnosis on families

Women continue to provide the majority of care for children. Fear of the children being removed from their care or lack of alternative, acceptable childcare provision may impact on a woman not accessing services for either her substance misuse or her mental health problems.

The Hidden Harm (Hidden Harm, A Report of an Inquiry by the Advisory Council on the Misuse of Drugs) report suggests that there are between 250,000 and 350,000 children of problem drug users in the United Kingdom – about one for every problem drug user. Up to 1.3 million children in the United Kingdom are affected by parental alcohol problems. If we accept that the percentage of substance misusers with a co-existing mental health problem is 50% (Hidden Harm & AHRSE 2004), this represents 1–4% of all children under 16 having at least one parent with a dual diagnosis. The Hidden Harm report also states that of problem drug users 37% of fathers and 64% of mothers are living with their children. It is estimated that between 50 and 90% of families on social workers' childcare caseloads have one or both parents with drug, alcohol or mental health problems (Kearney *et al.* 2003). Eighteen thousand children have a mother who is sent to prison each year and, as discussed later, most women entering prison have a diagnosable mental illness and/or substance misuse problem.

Children brought up in an environment of psychological instability and substance misuse are at risk of both physical and emotional neglect and are at greater risk of emotional, physical and sexual abuse. The perpetrator of the sexual abuse may not be the parent, but the abuse is more likely to go unnoticed by a parent distracted by their substance misuse and/or mental health problem. These children are also more likely to adopt maladaptive coping strategies such as substance misuse, criminal behaviour and self-harm, as well as psychological problems later in life.

CASE STUDY 3

As a child Susan had been placed in foster care due to the sexual abuse she suffered at the hands of both her father and paternal uncle. She self-reported having had behavioural problems during adolescence and early adulthood. By the time she came into contact with her local drug services, she had had several admissions to psychiatric services following episodes of self-harm and suicide attempts as well as two custodial sentences for burglary and criminal damage. She was in a relationship with a drug user who had fathered three of her five children, all of whom were in care. She continued to sex work in order to fund both her and her partner's drug use. Susan was difficult to engage, frequently turning up late for appointments or missing them altogether. She dropped out of treatment when her youngest child was formally adopted.

Of special consideration are pregnant women. The period around childbirth is the time when women are most likely to suffer a mental illness due to the effects of childbirth on a woman's physiological, social and psychological world and the subsequent life adjustments required in caring for a newborn baby (Kendall et al. 1987). In order to minimise any deterioration of their mental health or increase in substance use, women with a dual diagnosis around the time of childbirth will require multi-agency input in order to provide the support required. This support should be provided by mental health services and substance misuse services as well as by mid-wives and health visitors. Many antenatal clinics now have a specialist service for drug-using mothers to enable co-working, but for women with mental health problems service provision remains scarce.

Women with a dual diagnosis are more likely to have multiple sexual partners and are less likely to use birth control. Pregnancies are often unplanned and may be undetected until the pregnancy is well advanced. Many substance-misusing women believe themselves unable to conceive because of irregular menstrual cycles as a result of poor nutrition and low body weight. Chaotic drug and alcohol use during pregnancy can lead to miscarriage or birth defects or later behavioural difficulties for the children. The maternal mental health may deteriorate during pregnancy as prescribed medication for their mental ill health is reduced or withdrawn for the duration of the pregnancy because of risk of harm to the unborn child. This, in turn, may lead to an increase in unprescribed drug or alcohol use in an attempt to alleviate unwanted symptoms. Again a reluctance to attend statutory services because of concerns that their unborn baby will be taken from them may prevent women from accessing health care or from disclosing the extent of their substance misuse.

Dual diagnosis and domestic violence

Many women attending either mental health services or substance misuse services have suffered domestic violence. In the general population in the United Kingdom, the lifetime rate of women who have suffered domestic abuse is 26% (Walby and Allen 2004). This compares to studies that show that the women in substance misuse treatment agencies have suffered domestic abuse at a rate of between 40 and 62%. For women in custody, 50% report emotional or physical abuse (Humphreys *et al.* 2005). These reports focus on physical abuse, but when psychological abuse is taken into account these figures rise to 90–100% (Corston 2007).

Women attending both domestic violence services and mental health care services may report a similar range of symptoms, including symptoms of PTSD, low self-esteem, fear, anxiety and depression. Women are more likely to report domestic violence as a cause of these symptoms if directly asked (The Stella Project 2007), but even then may be unwilling to do so because of fear of reprisal from the perpetrator.

Of particular relevance to service providers is that alongside the high incidence of domestic violence victims among women in addiction treatment centres, half the men in the same centres reported being perpetrators of this type of violence (Galvani and Humphreys 2007). This uneasy mix of perpetrators and victims of abuse being treated at the same agency is likely to have an effect on retention rates and effectiveness of treatment. Staff need adequate training and confidence to be able to deal with this issue safely and effectively and to provide an environment where these issues, for both the men and women, can be addressed appropriately in order to improve the outcomes for the service users.

Dual diagnosis within the female prison service

Women in custody often present with the most complex of histories. They have been both the victims of crime (often physical or sexual abuse, either as a child or as an adult) and the perpetrators of crime. However, the crimes they commit are usually acquisitive, with only a small proportion committing violent crimes. They are likely to have mental health problems alongside a history of substance misuse. They may be involved in sex working, which carries a high risk of both physical complications such as HIV and other sexually transmitted diseases.

They are unlikely to have received adequate care and treatment for their substance misuse, mental or physical health problems. This may be due to a suspicion of health care services or simply that their chaotic lifestyles prevent them from accessing these services.

Women with a dual diagnosis are more likely than those without to come into contact with the criminal justice system. They are more likely to re-offend than other females. Their presentation is also different than men; women are less likely to commit violent crime and, while in prison, are less likely to be involved in violent incidents. However, the rate of self-harm and suicide acts is high. Females in custody are six times more likely to self-harm than men, and proportionally more women kill themselves than men, which is in direct contrast to figures of those not in custody (Corston 2007).

It has been reported that up to 80% of women in custody have diagnosable mental health problems and 75% have used illicit drugs in the 6 months before going into prison. Women whose criminal behaviour commenced before their drug use were more likely to have been victims of childhood sexual abuse. These same women were more likely to have diagnoses of personality disorder and to have problems with more than one substance.

In one study of females in custody, only 20% of the women who were intravenous drug users had attended drug treatment services (ONS 1997), and few were receiving help for their mental health problems.

The Corston report identifies the inadequate provision for women with mental health disorders while in custody and also questions the validity of custodial sentences for those who have not committed violent crime. Separation from children and other family members will contribute to the psychological distress of these women, as well as the breakdown of family relationships.

A case for gender-specific services

The presentation of women with a dual diagnosis differs significantly from that of men (Department of Health 2002). This can impact on providing effective treatment especially in a residential setting. As the ratio of men and women entering residential drug treatment is 3:1, women will usually be in a minority in a residential setting; thus, the bias will be towards the male clients.

Women are more likely than men to have child care responsibilities, so services should be tailored to provide a 'child friendly' approach, which may include provision for children, longer opening hours and flexibility in appointment times. Residential services that are able to admit children while their parents receive treatment should be accessible.

Women with substance misuse and mental health problems are likely to have suffered sexual, physical or emotional abuse, often from a male drug user; thus, mixed gender services may be perceived to be threatening environments for women, which will deter them from accessing such services. Even if they access these services, because of lack of alternative provision, they will be unlikely to disclose their issues of abuse.

These mixed gender services may also impact on the efficacy of treatment for the men, 50% of whom admit to be perpetrators of domestic violence. They will be less likely to admit this in an environment where the female victims of abuse are present.

An additional complication is that women with a dual diagnosis, especially those with borderline personality disorder, may exhibit seductive or sexualised behaviour. This behaviour is likely to continue in the residential unit, leading to the commencement of ill-advised relationships. During detoxification sexual desire often resurges, and relationships starting in residential treatment agencies are not uncommon. These relationships often lead to early discharge, either voluntary or enforced as the 'rules' of the treatment agency usually forbid sexual or exclusive relationships. This early discharge usually results in treatment not being completed and inadequate follow-up, which leads to relapse of their drug use, their mental health problems or both.

CASE STUDY 4
Jane, a 26-year-old crack and heroin user, with a diagnosis of borderline personality disorder was admitted to a residential, mixed gender service for detoxification with a plan to transfer to a residential rehabilitation programme once drug free. She was in a relationship with a male drug user, who was frequently violent towards her. During her time in treatment her partner would phone her at least three or four times a day, questioning her about the others who were in treatment with her. He began to accuse her of having a relationship with one of the males in treatment and threatened to assault her if she continued this perceived relationship. The situation became intolerable for Jane, and so she self-discharged before completing her detoxification.

Conclusion

Men and women have differing needs from substance misuse and mental health treatment services. There is still more stigma attached to women who misuse illicit substances, particularly if they have childcare responsibilities. These, in turn, may prevent them from accessing appropriate treatment. Studies have shown that there are many substance misusers with a co-existing mental health problem who do not access services at all and who are likely to end up in the criminal justice rather than the health care system.

To attain optimum mental and physical health, women with a dual diagnosis should be able to access gender-specific services. These should be readily accessible and able to offer flexibility in terms of attendance, with a low threshold for entering treatment. A care co-ordinator should be assigned to each client, ensuring that they receive the care relevant to all their needs. A 'one-stop shop' would be the ideal, where the client's mental health, addiction, physical health and social needs can all be addressed. This would encourage attendance with a more successful engagement with services and better treatment outcomes. Women should be able to access these services for as long as they feel they need to and have access to residential treatment services.

References

Alcohol Harm Reduction Strategy for England (AHRSE) (2004) London: Strategy Unit.

Califano JA Jr (2006) *Women under the Influence.* The National Centre on Addiction and Substance Abuse at Columbia University, Baltimore: The John Hopkins University Press.

Corston BJ (2007) *The Corston Report: A Review of Women with Particular Vulnerabilities in the Criminal Justice System.* London: The Home Office.

Department of Health (2002) *Dual Diagnosis Good Practice Guide.* London: DH Publications.

Galvani S, Humphreys C (2007) *The Impact of Violence and Abuse on Engagement and Retention Rates for Women in Substance Use Treatment.* London: National Treatment Agency.

Greenfield SF, Manwani SG, Nargiso JE (2003) Epidemiology of substance use disorders in women. *Obstetrics and Gynaecology Clinics of North America* 30 (3): 414–446.

Hidden Harms: *Responding to the needs of children of problem drug* (2003) Advisory Committee on the Misuse of Drugs. London: Home office.

Humphreys C, Regan L, River D, Thiara RK (2005) Domestic violence and substance use: tackling complexity. *British Journal of Social Work* 35: 1303–1320

Kearney P, Levin E, Rosen G (2003) *Alcohol Drug and Mental Health: Working with Families.* London: Social Care Institute for Excellence.

Kendall R, Chalmers J, Platz C (1987) Epidemiology of puerperal psychosis. *British Journal of Psychiatry* 150: 662–673.

Messina N, Wish E, Nemes S (2000) Predictors of treatment outcomes in men and women admitted to a therapeutic community. *American Journal of Drug and Alcohol Abuse* 26 (2): 207–218.

Moscato BS, Russell M, Zielezny M *et al.* (1998) Gender differences in the relation between depressive symptoms and alcohol problems: a longitudinal perspective. *American Journal of Epidemiology* 146: 966–974.

ONS (1997) *Survey of Psychiatric Morbidity among Prisoners in England and Wales.* London: Department of Health.

Stella Project Toolkit (2007) *Drugs Alcohol and Domestic Violence: Good Practice Guidelines.* London.

Turning Point and Rethink (2004) *Dual Diagnosis Toolkit.*

Walby S, Allen J (2004) *Domestic Violence, Sexual Assault and Stalking: Findings from the British Crime Survey.* Home Office Research Study, No. 76. London: Home Office.

Chapter 13

Drug-Induced Psychosis

Hülya Bilgin, Murat Soncul and Peter Phillips

Introduction

People presenting with psychotic symptoms with recent or concurrent use of drugs and/or alcohol are frequently seen in mental health services and often present a diagnostic conundrum: Are the symptoms entirely due to the recent use of substances (drug-induced psychosis)? Has the substance use triggered a relapse of a previously existing psychotic illness? Is the substance use an attempt at self-medication? Or has the substance use precipitated the onset of a first episode of psychotic illness? Poor understanding of the complex relationship between psychotic illness and substance use in this context can lead to misdiagnosis, elevated risk and management difficulties (Güleç & Köroğlu 1997; Poole & Brabbins 1996). The consequences of such misdiagnosis can be extremely serious, as seen in the case of Christopher Clunis who killed after his symptoms were wrongly attributed to drug use (instead of untreated schizophrenia) (Ritchie *et al.* 1994).

Dual diagnosis: a common problem

The prevalence of dual diagnosis is well documented in North American and European epidemiological studies, but less well described in other parts of the world. Largely, studies estimate prevalence between 10 and 50% of recent/current drug use in people with mental illness, although rates vary between community and in-patient studies and from those studies that exclude people with non-psychotic mental health problems. For example, in Germany, Soyka *et al.* (1993) reported a prevalence of 22% at the time of the first schizophrenic episode and 43% among people with chronic schizophrenia. In London, the reported rate of alcohol and substance use disorders is 49% for patients with mixed psychotic illnesses (Phillips & Johnson 2003). The comorbidity of schizophrenia and cannabis use is around

45% in Lebanon, whereas the lifetime rate of alcohol and drug use disorder in patients with chronic schizophrenia in Turkey is 13% (Altınay 2005).

After decades of research, it still remains very difficult to tease out the relationships between substance use and mental illness, in terms of the issues relating to the onset of mental illness and also of the issues surrounding drug use: since most substance use remains illegal, it is difficult to assess the quality and effect of substances and also to establish which substance had what effect. (Polydrug use is the most common pattern of drug use.) A number of experimental studies have produced evidence of transient psychotic symptoms, but these cannot really replicate substance use in community 'real-world' settings (Poole & Brabbins 1996).

The relationship between substance use and psychosis: aetiology

A possible explanation for the occurrence of co-morbid substance use and psychotic illness might be that substance use causes psychosis. The substances most discussed as candidates for an aetiological role in psychosis have been stimulants, cannabis and hallucinogens.

Cannabis is the most frequently investigated among substances that potentially lead to psychotic illness. The temporary psychotic condition related to cannabis use is called *acute toxic psychosis*. The term *cannabis psychosis* has been used in literature since last century (Danki *et al.* 2005) as a condition that can last a few days with hallucinations, delusions, loss of short-term memory and confusion, with a good response to treatment. This is discussed by Hughes in Chapter 14 in detail.

For amphetamine users, it has been suggested that up to 10% of chronic users develop a chronic psychotic disorder that lasts more than 6 months after remaining abstinent from amphetamine use (making it difficult to distinguish from chronic psychotic illness) and that abstinent amphetamine users may develop paranoid exacerbation after single doses of amphetamine (Yousef *et al.* 1995; Flaum & Schultz 1996). One of the few studies that has been longitudinal (McLellan *et al.* 1979) compared stimulant users (cocaine and amphetamine) with matched controls who were using depressant or narcotic substances. No subjects in any group demonstrated any psychotic phenomena on initial assessment. At later follow-up, a significant number of the stimulant users had developed chronic psychotic states, which again were indistinguishable from schizophrenia, but no such states had developed in the control group. These findings are not clear proof of the link, but could be consistent with the notion that schizophrenia has a multi-factorial aetiology in which genes, biology and environment interact; in this instance, substance misuse becomes the factor that projects the individual over a 'threshold' into a psychotic illness (Murray & Fearon 1999). The dopamine and opiate neurotransmission systems are biological hypotheses that become prominent in both schizophrenia and addictive behaviour. The structure of the hippocampus and the abnormalities of the frontal cortex facilitate reward mechanisms in schizophrenia consolidating the effects of substances while decreasing the control of repression over substance seeking behaviour (Dixon *et al.* 1990; Akvardar *et al.* 2003; Evren & Evren 2003). Homelessness, social isolation, poor interpersonal skills, poor cognitive abilities, failure at school/work, poverty, stigma of mental illness, failure with family, lack of structured daily activities and living in communities where drug use is common may increase the susceptibility of individuals with psychotic illness to certain influences and social trends that accompany drug use, which can increase the prevalence of dual diagnosis (Bachrach 1987; Dixon *et al.* 1991; Altinay 2005; Gibbins & Kipping 2006). The increased social approval of illicit drug use is often considered another potential environmental factor (Smith & Hucker 1994). Drug use can bring some motivation as it compensates for such risk factors. Socially isolated young people with poor social skills using drugs to be accepted in their local peer groups are examples of this model. They find themselves more socially acceptable and part of the peer community where substance use is a part of the social identity.

The potential role of newer 'recreational' drugs in the development of psychotic illness has been discussed recently. Although there have been some reports of psychotic illness occurring in association with ingestion of 3,4-methylenedioxymethamphetamine ('Ecstasy') (McGuire *et al.* 1994) or the stimulant plant leaf khat (Yousef *et al.* 1995), the development of psychotic symptoms in the context of use of these drugs does not appear to occur frequently enough to constitute evidence for a causal link, and the weight of evidence is not yet great enough to reach clear conclusions.

On the other hand, mental illness might increase the vulnerability to substance use disorders as drug use patterns are based on specific psychopharmacological effects rather than being coincidental (Altinay 2005; Gibbins & Kipping 2006). Changing undesirable mood conditions, alleviating intolerable anxiety and increasing the ability to cope with cognitive disabilities can be among the motivations behind substance use. According to Khantzian (1997), drug use is associated with their properties of compensation: the use of heroin to reduce feelings of aggression and anger and the use of cocaine to lift mood during depressive episodes are examples of this compensation (Dixon *et al.* 1990; Baigent *et al.* 1995; Akvardar *et al.* 2003; Yancar 2005). Although users are aware of long-term effects of specific drugs, their expectations are of the early effects such as the psycho-stimulant effect of nicotine compensating the cognitive disability increasing attention (Altinay 2005). Evidence of self-medication has been demonstrated by users who suggest that some drugs alleviate certain symptoms of their illness (although the hypothesis of self-medication is slightly controversial) (Evren & Evren 2003).

A model of relationships between psychotic illness and drug and alcohol use

It is, therefore, clear that the possible number of inter-relationships between substances, motivations for use and mental ill health states are extensive – and difficult to assess. In attempting to address this, Poole and Brabbins (1996) proposed a seven-point working model that expanded the descriptions of drug-related psychotic states offered in both the ICD-10 and the DSM-IV classification systems.

Intoxication that mimics functional psychotic illness
The direct pharmacological effect of the substance mimics the signs and symptoms of psychosis, established for stimulant drugs and cannabis. These states may persist for a number of days and can be dependent on drug half-lives.

Pathoplastic reactions in functional psychotic illness
Psychoactive substance use can change the clinical presentation in functional psychotic illnesses, so that, for example, schizophrenic symptoms may appear in affective illness subsequent to cannabis use.

Chronic hallucinosis induced by substance use
Alcohol hallucinosis and 'flashbacks' (recurrence of drug use experiences after cessation of use) in lysergic acid diethylamide (LSD) and cannabis use are caused by substance use, but persist even after lengthy periods of abstinence, having the properties of hallucinations (in that they are experienced as 'true' perceptions).

Drug-induced relapse of functional psychotic illness
Substance use directly produces the relapse of psychotic illness, with three possibilities: (1) patients may be 'self-medicating' symptoms of their illness with substances (therefore substance use is another symptom – not the cause of the relapse), (2) patients may be motivated to use substances when unwell as a result of impaired judgement and (3) use/intoxication may directly lead to relapse.

Withdrawal states
Delirium tremens (DT) is associated with alcohol withdrawal and is clearly very different than psychotic symptoms seen in individuals with functional psychotic illnesses (e.g. visual hallucinations and clouding of consciousness that might normally be expected in organic psychotic syndromes). DT has also been reported in benzodiazepine withdrawal.

Other reactions

Panic and extreme anxiety reactions are seen in hallucinogen and cannabis use and can be mistaken for psychotic symptoms. Post-intoxication depression is often seen in individuals who use stimulant substances and is sometimes referred to as *Monday blues* or *crashing*. As with any depressive condition, a risk for increased suicidality exists and should be assessed for. Confusional states with intoxication and clouding of consciousness occurs in individuals using a wide range of substances, and symptoms include hallucinations, paranoid ideas and agitation.

True drug-induced psychosis

This category refers to psychotic symptoms that occur in the context of drug use and can persist for a brief period after bodily elimination of the drug. The symptoms only recur in the context of further use of the substance by vulnerable individuals. Symptoms also subside on the administration of antipsychotic medicines and cessation of substance use.

CASE STUDY 1

Ben is a 28-year-old single Caucasian man living with his parents in a small English town. He is the youngest of six children (and the only one with any mental health problems). He attained average grades at school and passed normal developmental milestones. In his penultimate year at school, Ben's progress began to suffer, with poor school grades, and it became clear he was spending a lot of time with a small group of peers who were often in trouble for fighting and truancy and other conduct problems. At this time he began using substances, largely cannabis and amphetamine, which persisted through his teenage years into his adult life. He also used LSD and alcohol and cocaine occasionally, but never tried heroin or other narcotic substances (and never used through injection). His early adult life was characterised by poor quality of life, short relationships and difficulty gaining employment. He was arrested several times for intoxicated behaviour and fighting and at the age of 26 lost his driving license after a drunk driving charge. Shortly after this, his girlfriend at that time gave him an ultimatum about his substance use and their continued relationship, which Ben took very seriously. He planned to stop using speed and cannabis and to continue infrequent social drinking, much to the relief of his family and partner. Two months later, Ben for the first time began to express paranoid ideas, initially about his girlfriend (suspected of unfaithfulness), which quickly developed into a belief that his girlfriend (Emma) was having a sexual relationship with his father. A month later, Ben reported feeling that Emma was having a sexual relationship with the family pets (dogs) and was setting fires around the area of their house. Ben became almost completely preoccupied with these thoughts, and his parents reported he was unable to discuss anything else. After weeks of isolation, Ben's parents took him back to hospital, convinced he was using again – despite his denial of such use. Ben's urine drug screen revealed no use, and he confirmed he had not used for a period of 2–3 months when he was admitted. Ben was given a diagnosis of amphetamine-induced psychotic disorder with delusions. The intense quality of Ben's delusional ideas did not diminish after a week in hospital, and the ward team started to query whether Ben was actually suffering from a schizophrenic disorder. After 3 days, Ben began treatment with antipsychotic drugs. After a total of 6 weeks in hospital, Ben's delusional ideas were still present but he was less preoccupied with them. The past 2 years have been characterised by slow but steady improvements in Ben's mental state, although he still takes small doses of antipsychotic medicines.

Case study 1 key points

No family history of mental illness, conduct problems (school), criminal justice service involvement, frequent and heavy polydrug use, symptoms commonly associated with functional psychotic illness (but not hallucinations).

Conclusion

The above-mentioned case study demonstrates the diagnostic conundrum associated with patients presenting with this history and combination of symptoms and problems. In this case, the presenting features make understanding Ben's symptoms more straightforward than is often the case in clinical mental health services; however, the key points as outlined above might be seen in the presentation of a number of psychiatric or psychological syndromes, and it is critical to fully evaluate these possibilities before finalising Ben's diagnosis and subsequent treatment. A common clinical error is to assume that drug use and psychotic illness are causally associated in every case. As has been described above, substance use may well relate to an attempt at self-management of symptoms, or other reactions, and it is therefore appropriate to retain a critical perspective to the relationship between substance use and psychotic symptoms.

References

Akvardar Y, Tumuklu M, Alptekin K (2003) Schizophrenia and substance use. *Journal of Dependence* 4: 118–122.

Altınay CU (2005) The comorbidity of alcohol – substance use disorder in patients with schizophrenia and the effects of comorbidity on course of illness. Expertise thesis, Bakırköy Mental Health and Neurological Diseases State Hospital, Istanbul, Turkey.

Bachrach LL (1987) New directions for mental health services. *Leona Bachrach Speaks: Selected Speeches and Lectures* 35: 1–102.

Baigent M, Holme G, Hafner J (1995) Self-reports of the interaction between substance abuse and schizophrenia. *Australian and New Zealand Journal of Psychiatry* 29: 69–74.

Danki D, Dilbaz N, Okay T, *et al.* (2005) Atypical antipsychotic treatment in substance induced psychotic disorder: a review. *Journal of Dependence* 6: 136–141.

Dixon L, Haas G, Weiden PJ, *et al.* (1990) Acute effects of drug abuse in schizophrenic patients: clinical observations and patients' self-reports. *Schizophrenia Bulletin* 16 (1): 69–79.

Dixon L, Haas G, Weiden P, Sweeney J, Francis AJ (1991) Drug abuse in schizophrenic patients: clinical correlates and reasons for use. *American Journal of Psychiatry* 148 (2): 224–230.

Evren C, Evren B (2003) Comorbidity of alcohol-substance use disorders in schizophrenia: a review. *Turkish Journal of Psychiatry* 14 (3): 213–224.

Flaum M, Schultz SK (1996) When does amphetamine-induced psychosis become schizophrenia? *American Journal of Psychiatry* 153: 812–815.

Gibbins J, Kipping C (2006) Coexistent substance use and psychiatric disorders. In: Gamble C, Brennan G (eds). *Working with Serious Mental Illness: A Manual for Clinical Practice.* London: Elsevier.

Güleç C, Köroğlu E (1997) *Psikiyatri Temel Kitabı,* vol. 1. Ankara, Turkey: Hekimler Yayın Birliği.

Khantzian EJ (1997) The self-medication hypothesis of substance use disorders: a reconstruction and recent applications. *Harvard Review of Psychiatry* 4: 231–244.

McGuire PK, Cope H, Fahy T (1994) Diversity of psychopathology associated with use of 3,4 methylenedioxymethamphetamine. *British Journal of Psychiatry* 165: 391–395.

McLellan AT, Woody GE, O'Brien CP (1979) Development of psychotic illnesses in drug misusers: possible role of drug preference. *New England Journal of Medicine* 301: 1310–1314.

Murray RE, Fearon P (1999) The developmental 'risk factor' model of schizophrenia. *Journal of Psychiatric Research* 33 (6): 497–499.

Phillips P, Johnson S (2003) Drug and alcohol misuse amongst in-patients with psychotic illnesses in three inner-London psychiatric units. *Psychiatric Bulletin* 27 (6): 217–220.

Poole R, Brabbins C (1996) Drug induced psychosis. *British Journal of Psychiatry* 168: 135–138.

Ritchie J, Dick D, Lingham R (1994) *The report of the inquiry into the care and treatment of Christopher Clunis.* London: HMSO.

Smith J, Hucker S (1994) Schizophrenia and substance abuse. *British Journal of Psychiatry* 165: 13–21.

Soyka M, Albus M, Kathmann N, *et al.* (1993) Prevalence of alcohol and drug abuse in schizophrenic inpatients. *European Archives of Psychiatry and Clinical Neuroscience* 242 (6): 362–72.

Yancar C (2005) The evaluation of the effect of second axis comorbidity and personality features on dependence severity and quality of life in substance users. Expertise thesis, Bakirköy Mental Health and Neurological Diseases State Hospital, Istanbul, Turkey.

Yousef G, Huq Z, Lambert T (1995) Khat chewing as a cause of psychosis. *British Journal of Hospital Medicine* 54 (7): 322–326.

Chapter 14

Cannabis Use and Psychosis

Liz Hughes

Introduction

This chapter will consider cannabis, its effects on the brain and mental health and the emerging evidence for effective interventions for people with mental health problems. It will begin by exploring what cannabis is, how it acts on the body and the desired and less desired effects. Then the effects on mental health (as a factor in both the development of mental illness and the exacerbation of symptoms) will be explored with consideration of the recent epidemiological data on cannabis use and schizophrenia. Finally, recommendations and suggestions for approaches to care will be made based on current available evidence.

What is cannabis?

Cannabis (also known as marijuana, hashish, puff, blow and skunk) is derived from the Cannabis Sativa plant and is available in three forms in the United Kingdom:

- Cannabis resin (known as hash)
- Traditional herbal cannabis (known as marijuana), which is the dried plant
- Sinsemilla (including skunk), which is the dried plant

Cannabis resin is prepared from the flowering and other parts of the cannabis plant and is processed and compressed into hard dark brown/black blocks before being imported into the United Kingdom, mainly from North Africa. Traditional herbal cannabis is a dried plant preparation of flowers and leaves imported from the Caribbean, Africa or Asia, and sinsemilla is from the flowering tops of unfertilised female cannabis plants, which are produced by intensive indoor cultivation methods. Sinsemilla has high potency as it has high levels of active ingredients (or cannabinoids) (ACMD 2008).

How is it used?

Cannabis is mainly smoked, but can also be prepared in food or drinks. Users cut or crumble the resin into small pieces and roll it with tobacco and smoke it either as a 'joint' or in a 'bong'. A bong is a device designed so that cannabis smoke passes through water to cool it down and produces a more intense 'hit' of the drug as the smoke is inhaled. With inhalation the rate of intoxication can be managed as the effects are almost immediate, whereas if cannabis is eaten, the effects develop more slowly but may lead to greater intoxication than planned, as it is difficult to gauge how potent a cannabis cake will be.

Legal issues

Cannabis is an illegal drug under the 1971 Misuse of Drugs Act, which means that personal use, selling and trafficking are prohibited by law. Offenders face fines and possible prison sentences as a result of engaging in such activities. It is currently class C (which carries mild penalties) but is to revert to Class B following a decision by the UK government in May 2008. If someone is caught with small quantities of cannabis (for personal use), it is likely that they will just receive a warning or caution from the police. However, growing, preparing and selling large quantities will attract much more severe penalties (see Table 14.1). The issues of illegality are of particular concern for those working in in-patient facilities. Phillips and Johnson (2003) found that 52% of in-patients admitted smoking cannabis on the ward at least once in a 6-month period. The dual diagnosis guidance for in-patient and day hospitals has advice about how to manage drug use in these clinical areas (DH 2006b) and services should ensure that they have a policy related to this issue. According to the Misuse of Drugs Act 1971, it is illegal for an organisation or workers to knowingly allow drug use or dealing to occur in a unit that they have responsibility for and should take reasonable preventative steps. Community workers do not have the same legal accountability regarding issues of witnessing or knowing about minimal personal use if it is occurring in someone's own home or out in the street. However, if the activity is related to dealing, growing or preparing cannabis for sale, then they have a duty to report this to their team and the police. Workers should be clear about the limits of confidentiality and the legal situation in regards to cannabis use and ensure that the service users and carers are also aware of these. The NTA have produced guidance on this to assist and support workers manage these issues (NTA 2003).

How it affects the user

The effect of cannabis appears to result from the chemical component tetrahydrocannabinol (THC) and this binds to 'cannabinoid receptors' situated on the surface of cells in the brain, as well as elsewhere in the body. It works by

Table 14.1   Penalties associated with cannabis

Penalties for supply, dealing, production and trafficking
The maximum penalty is 14 years imprisonment. This has increased from 5 years for all class C substances including GHB and Valium. (The maximum penalty of 14 years' imprisonment is the same for Class B drugs.)

Penalties for possession
The maximum penalty was reduced from 5 to 2 years imprisonment in 2004, but it will return to 5 years if Parliament approves the reclassification to Class B

Young people in possession of cannabis
A young offender in possession of cannabis will be arrested and taken to a police station where they can receive a reprimand, final warning or charge depending on the seriousness of the offence

Following one reprimand, any further offence will lead to a final warning or charge. Any further offence following a warning will normally result in a charge being brought. After a final warning, the young offender must be referred to the Youth Offending Team to arrange a rehabilitation programme to prevent reoffending

Adults in possession of cannabis
It is unlikely that adults caught in possession of cannabis will be arrested. Most offences of possession result in a warning and confiscation of the drug. However, some instances may lead to arrest and possible caution or prosecution, including

- repeat offending;
- smoking in a public place;
- instances where public order is threatened and
- possession of cannabis in the vicinity of premises used by children.

(Source: Home Office http://www.homeoffice.gov.uk/drugs/drugs-law/cannabis-reclassification/)

mimicking the action of several naturally occurring neurotransmitter substances known as 'endocannabinoids'. THC, however, is only one of around 60 'cannabinoids' present in preparations of cannabis. The pharmacological properties of most of these are unknown. One particular cannabinoid that has attracted recent attention is cannabidiol (CBD). There is growing evidence that this may have antipsychotic properties, but the mechanism is yet unknown.

Psychological effects

Users report that cannabis use creates a feeling of euphoria, depersonalisation, somnolence (sleepiness), altered sensory and time perception and relaxation. In acute intoxication, there are some less desirable effects such as perceptual disturbances and cognitive and motor impairment in healthy individuals; it can exacerbate pre-existing symptoms of psychosis in those with schizophrenia. First time and inexperienced users have been known to have acute attacks of anxiety, panic and paranoia. This usually subsides after an hour or so and will not require treatment, but it does help if people receive support and reassurance to help cope with what can be quite an unpleasant experience. The increased flow occurs in areas of the brain associated with mood, and there is decreased blood flow to areas associated with attention. There is less evidence that cannabis alters brain structure, although some studies have demonstrated that grey and white matter is less dense in cannabis users. Acute and residual neuropsychological effects can last up to 24 hours and these include deficits in attention, executive functioning and short-term memory. Heavy cannabis use can impair processing speed and ability to focus attention, and ignore irrelevant information. These deficits last longer than the period of intoxication and seem to worsen with increasing years of use. In a meta-analysis of studies of long-term effects where they existed they seemed to be related to learning and memory.

Physical effects

Cannabis alters blood flow in the body, which results in dilatation of some blood vessels but constriction of others. The characteristic redness of the eye is due to this. Constriction of blood vessels, however, causes a rise in blood pressure, which can put strain on the cardiovascular system. Paradoxically, cannabis can disrupt the control of blood pressure, leading to a lower standing blood pressure and an increased risk of fainting when standing up. People with heart problems should avoid cannabis as it increases heart rate and may exacerbate an existing condition.

Safety issues

The main risks associated with cannabis are as follows:

- Accidents as a result of inattention and poor reaction times
- Mental health symptom triggered or exacerbated
- Cardiovascular problems
- Cancer of the mouth, throat and lungs, and lung disease (although this may be due to the fact that cannabis is frequently smoked with tobacco)

(See Talk to Frank DH (2006a) Cannabis Toolkit for more information.)

The links between cannabis and psychosis

Prevalence of cannabis among those with schizophrenia

Cannabis is the second most commonly used psychoactive substance after alcohol in the United Kingdom and is commonly used in other countries too (EMCDDA 2006). It is estimated that almost half of people in their twenties in the United Kingdom have used cannabis at least once in their lifetime, although it is less common in older groups. However, the vast majority of young people are not using regularly. When considering the previous month before survey was performed, the proportion of current users drops to between 10 and 20%.

The rates found in people with mental illness seem to reflect use in the general population. Condren *et al.* (2001) found that rates of substance misuse history in people with schizophrenia and healthy controls taken from a general practice in the same area of Dublin were about the same (at around 40%). There is variation in prevalence of cannabis in those with serious mental illness. Rathbone *et al.* (2008) summarise international studies with prevalence range from 5% (Germany; Soyka *et al.* 1993) to 69% (Sweden; Allebeck *et al.* 1993). In the United Kingdom, the lifetime prevalence (if someone has ever had problems with cannabis) in mental health service users tends to be around 20% (Duke *et al.* 2001; Menezes *et al.* 1996). However, when considering current problems this rate tends to drop; Weaver *et al.* (2001) found that 10% of an inner city London community mental health service caseload had a current or persistent cannabis misuse problem. This was rated by case managers and so may be an under-representation of the true level.

In specific samples, the rates can be higher. In an early intervention service (which typically serves younger males), Barnett *et al.* (2007) found that half of the sample had used cannabis. Phillips and Johnson (2003) found that 70% of a sample from an in-patient setting in inner London had used at least once in the past 6 months, and 51% had used daily for at least 2 of the last 6 months.

Cannabis is used by a proportion of people with psychosis, and the following section will consider what impact that use has on the development of mental illness and on outcomes. However, it can be difficult to draw conclusions about this as people will often not be using cannabis in isolation; they will be taking a range of other psychoactive drugs (such as over-the-counter medications, stimulants, excessive caffeine, nicotine and alcohol) as well as prescribed medication (Miles *et al.* 2003), which will all interact.

The following section will consider the evidence for a specific link between cannabis and serious mental illness (such as psychosis).

Drug-induced psychosis

It is well established that cannabis use can cause a temporary psychosis – 'cannabis-induced psychosis'. This is a temporary state brought on by intoxication and should remit within a few hours to a few days, often without specialist treatment. However, some people may go on to develop a psychotic illness. Arendt *et al.* (2005) found that out of patients treated for cannabis-induced psychotic symptoms between 1994 and 1999 ($n = 535$), 44% went on to develop a schizophrenia spectrum disorder. Being young and male was also associated with increased risk of schizophrenia. Those who had a history of cannabis use developed schizophrenia at an earlier age than those who had never smoked cannabis. This suggests that cannabis use may play a precipitating role in the development of schizophrenia. Barkus *et al.* (2006) found that healthy (non-psychotic) individuals who scored highly on schizotypy (personality traits linked to future development of schizophrenia) were more likely to have psychosis-like experiences and more unpleasant after-effects after smoking cannabis. This suggests that those more vulnerable to psychosis are more likely to experience these kinds of symptoms with cannabis.

Does cannabis use in adolescence lead to schizophrenia?

Findings of several epidemiological studies indicate that smoking cannabis in adolescence increases the risk of developing schizophrenia in later life. Andreasson *et al.* (1987) followed up Swedish army conscripts from age 18 onwards and found that those who admitted smoking cannabis in adolescence had an increased risk of being diagnosed with schizophrenia. It was also suggested that there is a dose–response relationship; in other words, the heavier the use and the younger the age of first use, the higher the risk of developing schizophrenia. In a more recent analysis of this data, Zammitt *et al.* (2002) found that heavy use of cannabis by age of 18 led to an increased risk of schizophrenia by a ratio of 6:7. However, controlling for other confounding factors (such as disturbed behaviours, low intelligence quotient (IQ), growing up in a city and poor social integration) decreased the impact of cannabis on the risk by over half to 3.1.

The Dutch NEMESIS study by van Os *et al.* (2002) examined cannabis use in the general population ($n = 4059$) and a group of people with psychotic illness ($n = 59$). They found that lifetime exposure to cannabis was an independent factor in the development of psychosis in a dose–response related manner in previously psychosis-free individuals. Among the users with no prior history of psychosis, cannabis was linked to developing symptoms in 50% of the users.

In the Dunedin health and birth cohort study in New Zealand (1037 people who were born between 1972 and 1973), Arseneault *et al.* (2002) found that after controlling for pre-existing psychotic symptoms and use of other drugs (such as amphetamines), cannabis use increased the risk of schizophrenia. They also found that the risk was greater if the onset of cannabis was early (<15 years old). One explanation for this is that adolescence is a critical time in brain development moving towards adulthood, and cannabis use at this time impairs or interferes with this process.

Miettunen *et al.* (2008) reported on a prospective birth cohort study in Finland. The children (aged 15–16 years) were assessed on cannabis use and prodromal symptoms of psychosis (PROD). The proportion of adolescents that had ever used cannabis was quite small, 5.6%, and only 0.9% had smoked more than five times. They found that those who had ever tried cannabis had a higher mean score on the PROD, and this remained significant after controlling for the following: early emotional and behavioural problems (assessed by teachers at the age of 8), gender, family type, social class, regular tobacco use, use of other drugs and parental substance use disorders. There may be other confounders that may be contributing to the association that have not been measured and controlled for. Because of such low numbers of users in this study, it is difficult to draw conclusions from this.

The findings of the epidemiological studies have generated a good deal of debate. Some authors believe that cannabis is a significant causal factor for schizophrenia, but some are more cautious in their interpretation. Arseneault *et al.* (2004) reviewed the epidemiological studies available at that point and concluded that cannabis use doubles the risk of later life schizophrenia, and if cannabis use was eliminated in the population, this would result in 8% less cases of schizophrenia. This is also echoed by Smit *et al.* (2004), although they note that when confounding factors are controlled for, the risk of developing schizophrenia does decrease. In a more recent review, Ben Amar and Potvin (2007) conclude that cannabis may be a contributing factor, but that there are still unresolved issues such as the possibility of 'residual confoundings' (factors that have not been measured and therefore cannot be controlled for in the analysis), reverse causality (that psychosis leads to cannabis use) and the variation in how psychosis and cannabis use is measured in the epidemiological studies.

In conclusion, cannabis use in adolescence increases the risk of development of schizophrenia, but this is fairly modest and does decrease significantly when other factors (which also predict schizophrenia) are controlled for. In addition, there may be other factors that are as yet uncontrolled for that is producing this statistical effect. However, until more definitive evidence to refute this is available, the consensus is that young people should be aware of both the mental and physical health risks associated with cannabis use and, therefore, be able to make an informed choice about whether to use or not.

Cannabis use exacerbates symptoms of psychotic illness

There is some evidence that cannabis exacerbates symptoms of psychosis and may precipitate relapse and re-hospitalisation. Linszen *et al.* (1994) found that symptoms of psychosis were much worse for a group of people with schizophrenia who smoked cannabis compared to those who did not. Hides *et al.* (2006) found that cannabis use was predictive of worsening symptoms even after controlling for effects of medication adherence, other substance use and duration of illness. Addington and Addington (2007) found that the use of cannabis was associated with increased positive symptoms in a sample from an early intervention service in Denmark. Degenhardt *et al.* (2007) found that recent (in the previous month) cannabis use by people with schizophrenia predicted a small but statistically significant increase in psychotic symptoms in the following month, but had no effect on depressive symptoms. They found no association between increased psychiatric symptom severity and cannabis use, and that cannabis use was more likely to occur after reporting less severe symptoms.

These studies seem to indicate that cannabis may exacerbate symptoms of psychosis, but it is difficult to tease out the independent effect cannabis is having compared to other exacerbating factors such as stress, social problems, non-compliance with medication and so on.

How does cannabis affect psychosis?

If we are to accept that cannabis has an effect on increasing the risk of developing psychosis and exacerbates symptoms of those already ill, then we need to explore the hypotheses as to the mechanism of this.

1. *Self-medication hypothesis*

This suggests that people with schizophrenia use cannabis to alleviate negative symptoms. However, this has not been borne out with research. Generally speaking, cannabis use seems to pre-date psychotic symptoms rather than the other way around. This also does not fit with service users' own experiences and reasons for use, which often revolve around issues of relaxation and euphoria and alleviation of boredom and social reasons rather than psychiatric symptoms. Green *et al.* (2004) examined the reasons for cannabis use in people with psychosis and those without psychosis and found that the motives were similar.

2. *Stress-vulnerability theory or interaction hypothesis*

This suggests that there is a complex interplay between underlying vulnerability factors (such as family background, genetic make-up and early development) and 'stress' factors (such as substance misuse, relationship and financial problems) that ultimately lead to development of a mental illness such as schizophrenia (Hambrecht & Hafner 2000). Cougnard *et al.* (2007) found that common non-clinical psychotic experiences seen in adolescence were more likely to be persistent (and lead to the development of schizophrenia) if there was more exposure to environmental risk factors such as cannabis use, childhood trauma and urbanicity (living in an urban environment). They suggest that there is a synergistic relationship between the risk factors, with the number of risks being greater, the higher the chances of long-term psychotic illness. The *COMT* gene has been associated with less efficient breakdown of dopamine (which is one of the neurotransmitters associated with psychotic symptoms), and this coupled with adolescent cannabis use may increase the risk of adult schizophrenia (van Winkel *et al.* 2008). The epidemiological data suggest that this may be a viable explanation, given that the use of cannabis at critical developmental stages such as adolescence may be an added stressor that could lead to the development of schizophrenia. On the other hand, cannabis may be merely a marker for poor adaptation and coping in adolescence, which is associated with later onset of psychotic illness.

3. *Neurophysiological changes*

The brain has an endogenous cannabinoid system that is thought to be involved in cognitive functioning, emotions and reward. Changes in this system have been reported in schizophrenia. Cannabis use can alter the functioning of this system and this may explain why use can lead to an emergence or exacerbation of psychotic symptoms.

Interventions for cannabis and psychosis

Generally speaking, there is limited evidence for effective interventions that specifically target cannabis use in those with mental illness. Most of the research targets all substance use. From the substance use treatment world, there is some encouraging evidence that brief motivational interviewing (MI) can reduce cannabis use in healthy adolescents (McCambridge & Strang 2004; Olmstead *et al.* 2007).

Approaches that show efficacy with substance using populations may need adaptation to be suitable for those people with dual diagnosis (Bellack *et al.* 2006; Carey *et al.* 2007). This will include taking into consideration attention span, cognitive deficits, effects of psychiatric symptoms and medication. MI adapted for people with serious mental illness has shown promise with medication issues (Kemp *et al.* 1996; Gray *et al.* 2004); however, the current evidence for the use of MI with dually diagnosed people is inconclusive.

Baker *et al.* (2002) evaluated the use of MI for substance use in psychiatric in-patient setting in a randomised trial of one session MI or one information-giving session. A significant proportion (66%) of the sample had cannabis abuse or dependence. They found a modest short-term effect of MI, but this was not sustained over a longer time period. Cannabis use in particular seemed unchanged at 12 months follow-up. They suggest that cannabis consumption remains fairly stable and they found no relation between levels of cannabis use and psychiatric symptoms. They recommended that people with mental health problems may need more than one session of MI to demonstrate an impact.

Martino *et al.* (2006) conducted a randomised pilot study of a two-session MI for people with psychotic and mixed drug-related disorders who were entering an intensive outpatient programme. They compared the efficacy of this with a two-session standard psychiatric interview over a 12-week follow-up period. They found that both interventions improved substance use and psychiatric outcomes. However, when they compared different drug-using groups, it seemed that the cocaine-using group did significantly better with the MI than the cannabis-using group. This may be because there are more immediate negative effects of using cocaine than cannabis, which may be drawn upon in the MI.

The findings from these studies suggest that although MI is acceptable for this group and demonstrates some promise, a more powerful longer term intervention may be required to assist people with complex needs to make sustainable changes. A number of studies have used more intensive longer term interventions that have combined MI with other psychosocial interventions that are modified for people with serious mental illness.

Barrowclough *et al.* (2001) demonstrated some effectiveness of a programme of family work, MI and cognitive behavioural therapy (CBT) for people with schizophrenia and substance use (mainly cannabis and alcohol); however, only 3 out of 36 participants used cannabis. The majority used both alcohol and other drugs. This study demonstrated improvement in general functioning, reduction in positive symptoms and an increase in the percentage of days abstinent from drugs or alcohol in the 12-month follow-up period. Bellack *et al.* (2006) found that a group programme (behavioural treatment for substance abuse in serious and persistent mental illness – BTSAS) consisting of harm reduction, social skills training, motivational enhancement and contingency management (offering rewards for abstinence) was more effective than a 'treatment as usual' supportive group in reducing levels of substance use.

Edwards (2006) compared a cannabis and psychosis intervention ('CAP' – based on CBT and MI) with psycho-education sessions following initial treatment for early intervention psychosis. They found no significant differences between the interventions; cannabis use decreased in both groups. It was unclear whether cannabis use decreased as part of a natural process of being in treatment or whether the specific interventions helped.

In a follow-up study to the one session MI trial (Baker *et al.* 2002), Baker *et al.* (2006) evaluated a longer intervention of ten sessions of MI and CBT compared with routine treatment for a group of community-based people with psychosis and hazardous use of alcohol, cannabis and/or amphetamines. They found a short-term trend in improvements in cannabis use in the intervention group, but this was not sustained at 12-months post-treatment. Overall, the intervention group showed better overall functioning, but there was no difference in substance use outcomes.

Kemp *et al.* (2007) conducted a randomised trial of 4–6 sessions of a tailored programme of CBT for co-morbid substance use (called *Stop Using Stuff*) compared with treatment as usual and found that those exposed to the active intervention significantly improved on both cannabis and alcohol outcomes.

The findings of these studies are encouraging, but it is unclear whether these types of interventions would be effective with a sub-group of people with psychosis who use only cannabis. In addition, it is unclear how these complex interventions could be delivered by practitioners providing routine care. This would require specialist training and on-going supervision. Because these studies used a range of interventions, it is also unclear what the 'active ingredient' is. For instance, is MI sufficient for change, or do people with dual diagnosis require interventions that target symptoms, cravings and urges, working with families and carers, etc. It may be that individuals will require an individually tailored package depending on their specific needs.

The main drug of choice in the BTSAS study was crack cocaine that tends to have a more immediate and negative effect on a person and this lends itself to MI strategies (such as pros and cons of use), whereas the negative effects of cannabis may be more subtle and long term. In light of this, Martino *et al.* (2006) suggest that there may be a place for a more directive non-MI approach that seeks to stop cannabis use by legal means and reduces access to social services if a person continues to use cannabis. The difficulty with taking this approach is that one needs to be certain that a person's mental health problems are being profoundly affected by their use of cannabis and also need to be sure that the reasons for continued use are identified and managed. This approach suggests that cessation of cannabis use will solve a lot of problems, but, in fact, it may not be the case. They may be more lonely (as they have lost their peer group who they smoked with), they may still have unpleasant symptoms and cognitive deficits and they will still have social problems such as accommodation, family problems, etc.

In considering the role of cannabis use for the individual, it is important to take a holistic view of that person's life and explore where cannabis fits into this. The reasons for starting and continuing use are important to examine as these can highlight areas for intervention. This could include difficulties relaxing, sleeping, socialising, boredom and looking for something fun to do. The reasons for use will need to be tackled before any attempt to reduce the use can occur. This also means that the persons themselves need to be motivated to want to change their use. This requires them recognising for themselves that cannabis causes more problems than it solves. We can help people to explore the option of reducing or stopping cannabis by offering advice and information on cannabis and mental health, exploring their experiences of the drug and offering alternatives. However, no intervention, however good, can make someone change. Workers need to accept this and accept the service user's choices whatever they may be.

Conclusion

Cannabis is a commonly used drug in the general population and also in the sub-group of people with psychosis (and other mental health problems). The reported reasons for use seem to be similar to general population (for fun, socialising, relaxation, etc.) as opposed to medicating symptoms of psychosis. There is some evidence that cannabis use in adolescence is related to an increased risk of developing psychosis; however, when controlling for other risk factors, the risk decreases. There is also evidence that cannabis use may exacerbate symptoms of psychosis for people diagnosed with schizophrenia. The adverse effects of cannabis are subtle and become apparent over the long term, rather than immediately, which means that users are often more aware of the pleasurable short-term effects (relaxation, slowing of thoughts and help with sleep). This means that it may take a long time for people to develop awareness that cannabis may be detrimental to their mental health. Interventions based on the principals of MI (empathy, non-judgment, acceptance and non-confrontational stance) may be useful in assisting an individual to consider their choice of using cannabis, weighing up the pros and cons of use. However, as with other psychosocial approaches, MI needs to be adapted to the needs of people with serious mental illness to compensate for the cognitive impairments, distracting symptoms and effects of prescribed medication that may affect the ability to retain information and reflect on it in a meaningful way.

It is also important not to get fixated on cannabis use as the main problem or cause of the person's illness. People with complex needs such as 'dual diagnosis' have complex reasons for their problems and these require a holistic and comprehensive response that cuts across social and health boundaries. Assisting someone to reduce or stop smoking cannabis without providing them with support and alternative coping strategies is always doomed to fail. We need to work with service users in a collaborative way towards the goals that they want to achieve, which initially may or may not be related to their cannabis use. We also need to offer advice and support to families and carers who may be extremely anxious and upset about their relative's use of cannabis and assist them in managing this issue in the home.

Finally, there is a need to develop research into the experience of cannabis in psychosis, to continue to develop an evidence base for interventions (such as MI and CBT) and to ensure that workers have the requisite attitudes and skills to deliver those interventions in partnership with service users and their carers.

References

Addington J, Addington D (2007) Patterns, predictors and impact of substance use in early psychosis: a longitudinal study. *Acta Psychiatrica Scandinavica* 115 (4): 304–309.

Advisory Council for Misuse of Drugs (ACMD) (2008) *Cannabis: Classification and Public Health*. London: Home Office. http://drugs.homeoffice.gov.uk/publication-search/acmd/acmd-cannabis-report-2008?view=Binary.

Allebeck P, Adamsson C, Engstrom A, Rydberg U (1993) Cannabis and schizophrenia: a longitudinal study of cases treated in Stockholm County. *Acta Psychiatrica Scandinavica* 88 (1): 21–24.

Andreasson S, Allebeck P, Rydberg U (1987) Schizophrenia in users and nonusers of cannabis. A longitudinal study in Stockholm County. *Acta Psychiatrica Scandinavica* 79 (5): 505–510.

Arendt M, Rosenberg R, Foldager L, Perto G, Munk-Jorgensen P (2005) Cannabis-induced psychosis and subsequent schizophrenia-spectrum disorders: follow-up study of 535 incident cases. *The British Journal of Psychiatry: The Journal of Mental Science* 187: 510–515.

Arseneault L, Cannon M, Poulton R, *et al.* (2002) Cannabis use in adolescence and risk for adult psychosis: longitudinal prospective study. *British Medical Journal* 325 (7374): 1212–1213.

Arseneault L, Cannon M, Witton J, Murray RM (2004) Causal association between cannabis and psychosis: examination of the evidence. *The British Journal of Psychiatry: The Journal of Mental Science* 184: 110–117.

Baker A, Bucci S, Lewin TJ, *et al.* (2006) Cognitive-behavioural therapy for substance use disorders in people with psychotic disorders: randomised controlled trial. *The British Journal of Psychiatry: The Journal of Mental Science* 188: 439–448.

Baker A, Lewin T, Reichler H, *et al.* (2002) Evaluation of a motivational interview for substance use within psychiatric in-patient services. *Addiction* 97 (10): 1329–1337.

Barkus EJ, Stirling J, Hopkins RS, Lewis S (2006) Cannabis-induced psychosis-like experiences are associated with high schizotypy. *Psychopathology* 39 (4): 175–178.

Barnett JH, Werners U, Secher SM, *et al.* (2007) Substance use in a population-based clinic sample of people with first-episode psychosis. *The British Journal of Psychiatry: The Journal of Mental Science* 190: 515–520.

Barrowclough C, Haddock G, Tarrier N, *et al.* (2001) Randomized controlled trial of motivational interviewing, cognitive behavior therapy, and family intervention for patients with comorbid schizophrenia and substance use disorders. *The American Journal of Psychiatry* 158 (10): 1706–1713.

Bellack AS, Bennett ME, Gearon JS, Brown CH, Yang Y (2006) A randomized clinical trial of a new behavioral treatment for drug abuse in people with severe and persistent mental illness. *Archives of General Psychiatry* 63 (4): 426–432.

Ben Amar M, Potvin S (2007) Cannabis and psychosis: what is the link? *Journal of Psychoactive Drugs* 39 (2): 131–142.

Carey KB, Leontieva L, Dimmock J, Maisto SA, Batki SL (2007) Adapting motivational interventions for comorbid schizophrenia and alcohol use disorders. *Clinical Psychology: Science and Practice* 14: 39–57.

Condren RM, O'Connor J, Browne R (2001) Prevalence and patterns of substance misuse in schizophrenia: a catchment area case–control study. *Psychiatric Bulletin* 25: 17–20.

Cougnard A, Marcelis M, Myin-Germeys I, *et al.* (2007) Does normal developmental expression of psychosis combine with environmental risk to cause persistence of psychosis? A psychosis proneness-persistence model. *Psychological Medicine* 37 (4): 513–527.

Department of Health (DH) (2006a) Cannabis Toolkit. http://www.csip.org.uk/national-programmes/national-programmes/national-insititute-for-mental-health-in-england/mental-health-and-cannabis.html.

Department of Health (DH) (2006b) *Dual Diagnosis in Mental Health Inpatient and Day Hospital Settings. Guidance on the Assessment And Management of Patients In Mental Health Inpatient and Day Hospital Settings Who Have Mental Ill-Health and Substance Use Problems.* London: Department of Health. http://www.dh.gov.uk/en/Publicationsandstatistics/Publications/PublicationsPolicyAndGuidance/DH_062649 (30.10.2006).

Degenhardt L, Tennant C, Gilmour S, *et al.* (2007) The temporal dynamics of relationships between cannabis, psychosis and depression among young adults with psychotic disorders: findings from a 10-month prospective study. *Psychological Medicine* 37 (7): 927–934.

Duke PJ, Pantelis C, McPhillips MA, Barnes TR (2001) Comorbid non-alcohol substance misuse among people with schizophrenia: epidemiological study in central London. *The British Journal of Psychiatry: The Journal of Mental Science* 179: 509–513.

Edwards J, Elkins K, Hinton M, *et al.* (2006) Randomized controlled trial of a cannabis-focused intervention for young people with first-episode psychosis. *Acta Psychiatrica Scandinavica* 114 (2): 109–117.

EMCDDA Statistical Bulletin (2006) European Monitoring Centre for Drugs and Drug Addiction. Available at: http://stats06.emcdda.europa.eu/en/home-en.html.

Gray R, Wykes T, Edmonds M, Leese M, Gournay K (2004) Effect of a medication management training package for nurses on clinical outcomes for patients with schizophrenia: cluster randomised controlled trial. *The British Journal of Psychiatry: The Journal of Mental Science* 185: 157–162.

Green B, Kavanagh DJ, Young RM (2004) Reasons for cannabis use in men with and without psychosis. *Drug and Alcohol Review* 23 (4): 445–453.

Hambrecht M, Hafner H (2000) Cannabis, vulnerability, and the onset of schizophrenia: an epidemiological perspective. *The Australian and New Zealand Journal of Psychiatry* 34 (3): 468–475.

Hides L, Dawe S, Kavanagh DJ, Young RM (2006) Psychotic symptom and cannabis relapse in recent-onset psychosis. Prospective study. *The British Journal of Psychiatry: The Journal of Mental Science* 189: 137–143.

Kemp R, Harris A, Vurel E, Sitharthan T (2007) Stop using stuff: trial of a drug and alcohol intervention for young people with comorbid mental illness and drug and alcohol problems. *Australasian Psychiatry: Bulletin of Royal Australian and New Zealand College of Psychiatrists* 15 (6): 490–493.

Kemp R, Hayward P, Applewhaite G, Everitt B, David A (1996) Compliance therapy in psychotic patients: randomised controlled trial. *British Medical Journal* 312 (7027): 345–349.

Linszen DH, Dingemans PM, Lenior ME (1994) Cannabis abuse and the course of recent-onset schizophrenic disorders. *Archives of General Psychiatry* 51 (4): 273–279.

Martino S, Carroll KM, Nich C, Rounsaville BJ (2006) A randomized controlled pilot study of motivational interviewing for patients with psychotic and drug use disorders. *Addiction* 101 (10): 1479–1492.

McCambridge J, Strang J (2004) The efficacy of single-session motivational interviewing in reducing drug consumption and perceptions of drug-related risk and harm among young people: results from a multi-site cluster randomized trial. *Addiction* 99 (1): 39–52.

Menezes PR, Johnson S, Thornicroft G, *et al.* (1996) Drug and alcohol problems among individuals with severe mental illness in south London. *The British Journal of Psychiatry: The Journal of Mental Science* 168 (5): 612–619.

Miettunen J, Tormanen S, Murray GK, *et al.* (2008) Association of cannabis use with prodromal symptoms of psychosis in adolescence. *The British Journal of Psychiatry: The Journal of Mental Science* 192 (6): 470–471.

Miles H, Johnson S, Amponsah-Afuwape S, *et al.* (2003) Characteristics of subgroups of individuals with psychotic illness and a comorbid substance use disorder. *Psychiatric Services* 54 (4): 554–561.

National Treatment Agency (NTA) (2003) *Confidentiality and Information Sharing.* http://www.nta.nhs.uk/publications/documents/nta_confidentiality_and_info_sharing_2003_dsp1.pdf.

Olmstead TA, Sindelar JL, Easton CJ, Carroll KM (2007) The cost-effectiveness of four treatments for marijuana dependence. *Addiction* 102 (9): 1443–1453.

Phillips P, Johnson S (2003) Drug and alcohol misuse among in-patients with psychotic illnesses in three inner London psychiatric units. *Psychiatric Bulletin* 27: 217–220.

Rathbone J, Variend H, Mehta H (2008) Cannabis and schizophrenia. *Cochrane Database of Systematic Reviews* 3 (3): CD004837.

Smit F, Bolier L, Cuijpers P (2004) Cannabis use and the risk of later schizophrenia: a review. *Addiction* 99 (4): 425–430.

Soyka M, Albus M, Kathmann N, *et al.* (1993) Prevalence of alcohol and drug abuse in schizophrenic inpatients. *European Archives of Psychiatry and Clinical Neuroscience* 242 (6): 362–372.

Talk to Frank (web-based information). Too Much Too Often. Guide to cutting down Cannabis. http://www.talktofrank.com/cannabis.aspx.

van Os J, Bak M, Hanssen M, *et al.* (2002) Cannabis use and psychosis: a longitudinal population-based study. *American Journal of Epidemiology* 156 (4): 319–327.

van Winkel R, Henquet C, Rosa A, *et al.* (2008) Evidence that the COMT (Val158Met) polymorphism moderates sensitivity to stress in psychosis: an experience-sampling study. *American Journal of Medical Genetics. Part B, Neuropsychiatric Genetics* 147B (1): 10–17.

Weaver T, Rutter D, Madden P, *et al.* (2001) Results of a screening survey for co-morbid substance misuse amongst patients in treatment for psychotic disorders: prevalence and service needs in an inner London borough. *Social Psychiatry and Psychiatric Epidemiology* 36 (8): 399–406.

Zammit S, Allebeck P, Andreasson S, Lundberg I, Lewis G (2002) Self reported cannabis use as a risk factor for schizophrenia in Swedish conscripts of 1969: historical cohort study. *British Medical Journal* 325 (7374): 1199.

Chapter 15

Methamphetamine and Mental Health

Melinda Campopiano

Introduction

Methamphetamine (MA) is so routinely associated with the clause 'a highly addictive drug' in the professional and lay literature that it is easy to conclude that it is more addictive than amphetamine or other drugs of abuse. The mechanisms of action and effect of MA are only subtly distinct from amphetamine (Sulzer *et al*. 2005). Both agents raise the levels of available dopamine, norepinephrine and serotonin by multiple molecular mechanisms (Barr *et al*. 2006). MA dissolves easily in fat, so it readily crosses the blood–brain barrier, making its effects felt more quickly than cocaine. It is eliminated from the body more slowly, causing it to last three or four times longer than cocaine (Barr *et al*. 2006). Unlike cocaine MA can be produced locally from readily available pharmaceutical, industrial and agricultural chemicals, potentially divorcing it from usual supply and distribution routes although precursor control has reduced local small-scale production in recent years (US Drug Enforcement Administration 2007). The reputation of MA as a particularly dangerous scourge is likely because its abuse has appeared in waves since the commercial introduction of the first amphetamine in the 1930s (Sulzer *et al*. 2005). It generally comes as a surprise to people familiar only with contemporary MA misuse that amphetamine, MA and methylphenidate are still widely prescribed for weight loss, narcolepsy, attention-deficit disorder and depression (Anglin *et al*. 2000; Sulzer *et al*. 2005).

MA is potent, long acting and cheap, making it a good value for the person determined to pursue its effects. According to the 2006 National Survey on Drug Use and Health, there are an estimated 731,000 current users of MA in the United States, a number that has been essentially stable since 2002. MA use shows a strong regional preference for the Western United States, where 1.6% of the population over age 12 reports use in the last year in contrast to 0.3% in the Northeast, where it is more a club or party circuit drug, and

0.5–0.7% in the Mid-west and South, respectively. According to this survey, twice as many men as women use MA.

CASE STUDY 1: ANGIE – A CASE STUDY IN RISK AND PROTECTIVE FACTORS

Angie, a white female, was born in Des Moines Iowa in 1962. She was the first born child of high-school-educated parents. Her father, a car salesman, and her mother, a homemaker, eloped to a nearby state in order to marry without parental consent when her mother was 18 and her father 20. Neither family supported the relationship, but the fact that both were devoutly Catholic required the couple to marry in the Church before living together. Angela's early childhood was characterised by parental immaturity, lack of financial means and marital discord. A sister was born in 1965. Angie was an active and talkative child who did above average work in her early school years and participated in after-school social and sporting activities. At the age of 10, she was molested by a teenage male family member and his friend but did not disclose this until mid-life. After this event, she began suffering from anxiety and panic attacks, which were looked upon as a behaviour problem. Angie's parents' financial circumstance improved slightly and the family relocated to a larger home when Angie was 13, causing her to enter seventh grade at a junior high school without her cohort of pupils from elementary school. She tolerated this social dislocation with difficulty but eventually adapted to the new school. Her parents divorced 3 years later, causing Angie, her mother and sister to move to a suburban apartment. Angie then enrolled as a tenth grader (age 16) in a large and affluent high school with students in grades 9–12. Her mother now required to work and Angie had minimal parental supervision and was expected to look after her younger sister. The divorce prompted her mother to abandon the Catholic Church. Angie's mother began dating and socialising with other adults. She began to permit alcohol to be stored in the home and disclosed to Angie that she experimented with marijuana.

Around this time Angie was diagnosed with anxiety and prescribed valium by her paediatrician. She experimented with misusing this medication but found it too sedating. Angie found social acceptance, formed close friendships and began having sexual encounters among high-school-age adolescents not enrolled in school, some of whom had older siblings who were employed and provided the younger teens with alcohol and marijuana. She shop-lifted small clothing items and make-up and once ran away with a girlfriend to Kansas City only to return after a few days. She no longer participated in school-related social functions or sports. She ultimately left school a few months before she would have received her diploma because she feared she would have to take summer classes and she preferred to look for work in order to have money and live with her friends. She quickly abandoned the use of alcohol as a mood-altering substance owing to its depressant effects. For a brief period after leaving school, she moved to Peoria with a boyfriend but returned when the relationship ended. During this time, she was introduced to MA as 'Biker's Coffee'.

At the age of 19 she married and became pregnant. Her marriage would not survive the stress related to the diagnosis and treatment of her newborn daughter's cancer. At the age of 22 she gave birth to a healthy son and remained married to the father of this child for several years despite regular episodes of physical abuse. She primarily worked as a waitress where her energetic and friendly personality was rewarded. She used MA on a regular weekly to monthly basis during this time in order to have energy to look after her family and socialise after working long shifts and for weight control. During her pregnancies and childbirth, Angie abstained from drug use and never disclosed her history of use to her obstetrician. She was never asked about drug use and neither she nor her children were ever tested. Angie and her children progressed through various domestic situations, sometimes living in a single room. Angie would allow her daughter's father to assume custody of the child in her early grade school years but kept custody of her son into his early adolescence. Her son would then go live with his father who also used MA and was involved in drug production and sales.

Initiation and continuation of methamphetamine use: missed opportunities

Initiation of drug use among adolescents is associated with individual, familial and social factors. According to the National Survey on Drug Use and Health, a young person's perception of parental and peer disapproval of substance use, religiosity and parental involvement in school and home life are protective against both licit and illicit substance use. Initiation into MA and other 'hard' drugs is associated with mental health treatment utilisation, licit substance and marijuana use, high sensation seeking and family disruption (Herman-Stahl *et al.* 2006). Females are more likely to be introduced to MA by a male partner (Herman-Stahl *et al.* 2006), but the use of MA for both males and females typically occurs within 'private domestic contexts, both family and acquaintance relationships' (Sommers 2006). Epidemiologic data indicate that among adult MA users 'three-quarters or more initiate their use of the drug while still in their teens, with more than a quarter beginning use before the age of 15' (Gibson *et al.* 2002). Much emphasis has been placed on the social and demographic differences between the poor, white, rural MA user and the party circuit user, but the commonalities between the motivations and risks for initiation to MA use would seem to indicate that social diffusion strategies for drug use prevention and harm reduction would be effective given appropriate communication strategies for each group (Gibson *et al.* 2002; McCaughan *et al.* 2005; Thorberg & Lyvers 2006).

Regular adult users of MA are often motivated to continue use to cope with mental distress, maintain alertness, suppress appetite and enhance sexual experience (von *et al.* 2002). Weight loss is a motivator for ongoing MA use among females more than among males (Herman-Stahl *et al.* 2006). Rural users appear to be at high risk for medical and psychiatric comorbidity due to earlier use, more frequent use by injection and more cigarette and alcohol consumption (Grant *et al.* 2007). Of rural Ohio adult MA users surveyed, most believed staying healthy was important but 41.3% indicated they felt their health was fair or poor. Unfortunately, 73.9% reported having no health insurance (Siegal *et al.* 2006), a number that is likely consistent across the rural United States. MA users are more likely than heroin users to be human immunodeficiency virus (HIV) infected because of having more sexual partners (Gibson *et al.* 2002) and engaging in higher risk sexual activity (Springer *et al.* 2007; Zule *et al.* 2007). MA users with HIV are less likely to adhere to HIV medication because of MA-related disruption of diet and sleep (Reback *et al.* 2003) and may derive less effect from anti-retroviral therapy due to direct interference from the MA itself (Ellis *et al.* 2003). The greater need for medical and psychiatric care among MA users combined with limited availability of such care in rural areas and poor access to these services paints an ugly picture of the health and future of rural MA users.

Screening and brief intervention by physicians and other health professionals across all health-care settings has been shown to be effective in identifying and reducing substance use disorders and improving utilisation of specialised treatment (Miller *et al.* 2006; Academic ED SBIRT Research Collaborative 2007). One study of brief intervention with MAs shows that the intervention resulted only in a reduction in number of days MA is used (Srisurapanont *et al.* 2007), but the benefit of this should not be discounted. Outreach and education about substance abuse treatment and risk reduction on the level of a public health intervention using appropriate social diffusion strategies (Sexton *et al.* 2006), in addition to screening and brief intervention at all health-care delivery points, can improve this population's access to treatment and reduce the personal and social harms related to MA use (Miller *et al.* 2006). Directly observed therapy may improve mental health treatment as well as HIV or Hepatitis C virus (HCV) treatment for MA users who can be engaged in community- or treatment-based programs (Kresina *et al.* 2004). Owing to the higher rates of HIV infection and other medical and psychiatric comorbidities, comprehensive case management (Copeland & Sorensen 2001; Cretzmeyer *et al.* 2003) may be of particular benefit.

Pregnant women, even adolescents, seem to be able to cease or curtail illicit substance use (Hall *et al.* 1993). In geographic areas and populations where MA use is high, one can reasonably expect to detect MA in a large portion of persons presenting for medical care (Bailey 1987), but this does not necessarily carry over into the pregnant population (Buchi *et al.* 2003; US Department of Health and Human Services 2007). The factor most predictive of an MA-positive toxicology result in a pregnant woman is self-reported history of substance use (Gurnack & Paul 1997), which suggests again that screening and intervention at the time of medical or social service encounter is a promising way to promote effective intervention on behalf of both mother and child. In 2005, the National Toxicology Program Center for the Evaluation of Risks to Human Reproduction (NTP-CERHR 2005) published its report on the reproductive and developmental toxicity of amphetamine and MA. The panel concluded that there is 'concern with regard to potential neurobehavioral alterations due to prenatal MA exposure in humans both in therapeutic and non-therapeutic settings' (NTP-CERHR 2005) and 'some concern' regarding amphetamines. Most human and animal data were judged inadequate to draw solid conclusions for a variety of reasons. Some studies were insufficiently powered to detect deformities, whereas others were not adequately controlled. Animal experiments used inappropriate species or routes of delivery among other problems (NTP-CERHR 2005). Further research into low birth weight and shortened gestation, the areas of greatest suggestive findings, is needed. Children of MA-using parents may be exposed to toxins in the course of MA production (Mecham & Melini 2002) and are at risk for neglect and emotional or behavioural disturbance due to their exposure to drug use behaviours, ineffective parenting and violence (Mecham & Melini 2002; Derauf *et al.* 2007). Interpersonal violence is reported by up to 80% of female MA users (Cohen *et al.* 2003) and puts the children at additional risk.

Angie spent the greater part of the 1990s actively involved in MA use. She became intimately linked to increasingly violent and more criminally involved men until she was arrested herself. She was sentenced to 10 months incarceration in a treatment unit of the state women's penitentiary. She was released to supportive housing only to relapse in order to fit back into her clothes. A couple of years later, she was imprisoned for 6 months on fraud and theft charges. She was paroled to an apartment owned by her father. She again relapsed in part to lose the weight she had gained in prison. With a felony record, she was unable to find gainful employment and for a period of several years surrendered herself completely to her drug use. For a time she provided shelter to a family friend who could not sleep in his own home because he was using the location to manufacture MA. She received drugs in exchange for this service. Angie was hospitalised on one occasion for skin and soft tissue infection, requiring intensive care management and suffered nerve damage to her leg after a botched injection. She was introduced to safer injection techniques via harm reduction literature sent to her without comment by her sister and began to disseminate this information among her peers. She credits learning these skills and the respect accorded her by other drug users with allowing her to develop some sense of choice and control with regard to her drug use. Some of her desires to abandon MA use derive from this period. Unfortunately, while on probation she attempted to introduce marijuana into the state prison to deliver to her then husband, a man she had married only to obtain the right to visit in prison, as felons are otherwise prohibited from visitation. For this charge she was ordered to serve two consecutive 5-year sentences. She had become active nationally in harm reduction activities as a user advocate and with the support of harm reduction advocates, and her family would appeal the decision and ultimately receive probation in 2005.

Methamphetamine and mental health: intoxication, withdrawal and psychiatric illness

MA use produces euphoria and increases energy alertness and libido. These symptoms are replaced with hypersomnia and dysphoria as the drug's effects wear off (Winslow *et al.* 2007). Regular MA use is not associated with the development of tolerance to the subjective effects of euphoria (Perez-Reyes *et al.* 1991), so escalation of use is more likely attributable to the psychological reward of use and to drug availability (Sommers 2006). Large doses or repeated use in a short period of time may elevate blood pressure, body temperature and heart rate, potentially leading to muscle breakdown, kidney failure, heart attack or stroke. Psychological consequences of excessive use include anxiety, paranoia and psychosis. In one survey of MA users, three quarters of respondents reported daily use with nearly all, engaging in periodic binge behaviour; however, 20% reported stable use over a period of many years. Those persons experiencing the greatest social and psychological harms reported the most frequent use. A substantial number of respondents reported experiencing little or no harmful consequences of their MA use (Sommers 2006).

Great care should be taken to distinguish between lingering acute intoxication or MA withdrawal and either mania or depression. The dysphoria and hypersomnia of MA withdrawal will be most intense for the first 24 hours, decrease steadily for 7–10 days but persist in milder form for 2 weeks or more after the initial withdrawal period. The withdrawal course can be expected to be longer and more intense for persons with a longer history of MA use (Newton *et al.* 2004; McGregor *et al.* 2005). There is no specific pharmacotherapy for the management of uncomplicated MA withdrawal (Kosten & O'Connor 2003; Winslow *et al.* 2007), but this period represents an important opportunity for intervention. Significant symptoms persisting more than a week after the acute withdrawal phase should be treated (Kosten & O'Connor 2003).

The prevalence of mental illness in all adults and particularly among substance using adults makes mental health treatment an essential partner of any substance abuse treatment intervention (US Department of Health and Human Services 2007). Serious psychological distress and major depressive episode are strongly predictive of initiation, continuation and relapse of substance use disorder (Thorberg & Lyvers 2006; US Department of Health and Human Services 2007). When compared to cocaine users, MA users have higher rates of psychiatric illness, ranging from major depression and bipolar disorder to anxiety disorders and post-traumatic stress (Copeland & Sorensen 2001). They also report a statistically significant higher number of past suicide attempts (Copeland & Sorensen 2001). Mood disturbance and anxiety appear to be most strongly associated with independent psychiatric diagnoses rather than with MA use (Vik 2007). Fluoxetine, imipramine and bupropion have shown some promise in reducing cravings and improving treatment compliance (Winslow *et al.* 2007) and should be considered for the treatment of anxiety or depression in the MA user. Smoking cessation may reduce triggers for relapse and improve overall health (Kosten & O'Connor 2003).

The incidence of psychosis among MA users is estimated by some to be up to 11 times greater than in the general population (McKetin *et al.* 2006), although some of this increase can be attributed to premorbid personality types and pre-existing mental illness that is more common in persons with substance use disorders (Chen *et al.* 2003; Simons *et al.* 2005; McKetin *et al.* 2006). A typical psychotic episode will last only hours and feature hallucination and paranoia. More severe cases will completely resolve within a week of cessation of MA use. Psychosis may recur with or without resumption of MA use and may be triggered by stress (Barr *et al.* 2006). The duration and amount of MA use are positively associated with an increased risk of psychosis (Chen *et al.* 2003).

A good deal has been said of the neurotoxic effects of MA use (Cho & Melega 2002; London *et al.* 2004; Sulzer *et al.* 2005), but this information is of limited clinical usefulness. Little is known about the premorbid brain morphology and neurobiology of MA users compared to either the general population or other drug users, making it impossible to distinguish between the results of MA use and naturally occurring but abnormal phenomena that may predispose to addiction (Simons *et al.* 2005; Barr *et al.* 2006; Thorberg & Lyvers 2006). MA users who have experienced psychosis 'are treated with anti-psychotic drugs, which have well established effects on brain morphology' (Barr *et al.* 2006), making some of the changes observed potentially iatrogenic in nature. The cognitive impairment associated with long-term MA use, particularly in attention and decision making, appears to be real (Barr *et al.* 2006), but only difficult-to-conduct prospective studies on reliably abstinent former long-term users will allow this to be borne out.

Methamphetamine addiction: treatment and outcomes

The treatment of MA use is primarily an outpatient endeavour and outcomes can be expected to be on par with the treatment of cocaine abuse (Copeland & Sorensen 2001; Luchansky *et al.* 2007). Results of a large naturalistic study published in 2006 by Brecht *et al.* identifies pre-treatment,

treatment-related factors and their associated outcomes up to 24 months after the treatment exposure. According to Brecht's results, any treatment for MA use is associated overall with less MA use and less criminal activity 24 months after the exposure (Brecht *et al.* 2006). Pre-treatment factors such as higher level of education, employment and absence of criminal activity increase the likelihood of reduced MA use and reduced criminal activity for a given individual during the 24 months after treatment (Brecht *et al.* 2006). Residential treatment, a higher degree of pre-treatment MA-related harm and lower pre-treatment MA use also predict less MA use in the 24 months after treatment. Coerced treatment is associated with greater likelihood of relapse within 6 months but is also frequently the first exposure to residential treatment and the longest period of treatment for a given individual (Brecht *et al.* 2005). MA users who inject have poorer treatment outcomes when compared to non-injectors (Rawson *et al.* 2007). Cognitive behavioural therapy and contingency management, whether conventional or manualised as in the matrix model, have the strongest evidence supporting their use with MA addiction (Herrel *et al.* 2000; National Institutes of Health 2006; Roll 2007), although 12-step-based interventions show promise (Donovan & Wells 2007). Female MA users report low self-worth, negative emotions, difficulty severing contacts with MA users and establishing relationships with non-drug users at least in part due to intimate relationships with male MA users and a lack of relapse prevention skills, all of which perpetuate the continuum of MA (Sun 2007). Such findings suggest that women may require more extensive social and interpersonal support in addition to traditional mental health and substance abuse treatment. There is no published data describing the extent or effects of childhood sexual abuse among female MA users.

Angie continues to serve her probation but now works to support herself and owns a car. She is receiving regular mental health care and is working to repair her relationships with her now grown children. She was recently diagnosed with hepatitis C. She credits the concepts of harm reduction for allowing her to take control of her drug use and behaviours. She presently has government-funded medical insurance and is receiving individual therapy and bupropion, which she finds helpful. She also attends outpatient treatment ordered by the court. She will likely lose her medical insurance soon because of the income she is generating by working full-time and it is questionable whether she will be able to afford her treatment once this coverage is ended.

Conclusion

Angie's case illustrates the series of missed opportunities that is the natural history of MA use. Stigmatised along with all substance use and subject to hyperbolic media coverage, MA use and the burden of mental illness that accompanies it are a public secret in American communities large and small. The lack of treatment resources is magnified by the failure to identify substance use disorders and the mental illness that makes spontaneous remission unlikely even when these conditions present in obvious and identifiable ways across a range of medical and public health settings. Non-judgmental screening followed by harm-reduction-based brief intervention can not only allow the MA user to access treatment but also to remain engaged in supportive programs that foster the adoption of lower risk behaviours associated with better long-term outcomes (Miller *et al.* 2006; Toumbourou *et al.* 2007).

Acknowledgements

The author wishes to thank her sister Angela for her help in developing the case study for this chapter.

References

Academic ED SBIRT Research Collaborative (2007) The impact of screening, brief intervention, and referral for treatment on emergency department patients' alcohol use. *Annals of Emergency Medicines* 50 (6): 699–710, 710.e1–710.e6.

Anglin MD, Burke C, Perrochet B, Stamper E, Dawud-Noursi S (2000) History of the methamphetamine problem. *Journal of Psychoactive Drugs* 32 (2): 137–141.

Bailey DN (1987) Amphetamine detection during toxicology screening of a university medical center patient population. *Journal of Toxicology–Clinical Toxicology* 25 (5): 399–409.

Barr AM, Panenka WJ, MacEwan GW, *et al.* (2006) The need for speed: an update on methamphetamine addiction. *Journal of Psychiatry and Neuroscience* 31 (5): 301–313.

Brecht ML, Anglin MD, Dylan M (2005) Coerced treatment for methamphetamine abuse: differential patient characteristics and outcomes. *American Journal of Drug and Alcohol Abuse* 31 (2): 337–356.

Brecht ML, Greenwell L, von Mayrhauser C, Anglin MD (2006) Two-year outcomes of treatment for methamphetamine use. *Journal of Psychoactive Drugs* (Suppl. 3): 415–426.

Buchi KF, Zone S, Langheinrich K, Varner MW (2003) Changing prevalence of prenatal substance abuse in Utah. *Obstetrics & Gynecology* 102 (1): 27–30.

Chen CK, Lin SK, Sham PC, *et al.* (2003) Pre-morbid characteristics and co-morbidity of methamphetamine users with and without psychosis. *Psychological Medicine* 33 (8): 1407–1414.

Cho AK, Melega WP (2002) Patterns of methamphetamine abuse and their consequences. *Journal of Addictive Diseases* 21 (1): 21–34.

Cohen JB, Dickow A, Horner K, *et al.* (2003) Abuse and violence history of men and women in treatment for methamphetamine dependence. *American Journal on Addictions* 12 (5): 377–385.

Copeland AL, Sorensen JL (2001) Differences between methamphetamine users and cocaine users in treatment. *Drug and Alcohol Dependence* 62 (1): 91–95.

Cretzmeyer M, Sarrazin MV, Huber DL, Block RI, Hall JA (2003) Treatment of methamphetamine abuse: research findings and clinical directions. *Journal of Substance Abuse Treatment* 24 (3): 267–277.

Derauf C, LaGasse LL, Smith LM, *et al.* (2007) Demographic and psychosocial characteristics of mothers using methamphetamine during pregnancy: preliminary results of the infant development, environment, and lifestyle study (IDEAL). *American Journal of Drug and Alcohol Abuse* 33 (2): 281–289.

Donovan DM, Wells EA (2007) 'Tweaking 12-Step': the potential role of 12-Step self-help group involvement in methamphetamine recovery. *Addiction* 102 (Suppl. 1): 121–129.

Ellis RJ, Childers ME, Cherner M, *et al.* (2003) Increased human immunodeficiency virus loads in active methamphetamine users are explained by reduced effectiveness of antiretroviral therapy. *Journal of Infectious Diseases* 188 (12): 1820–1826.

Gibson DR, Leamon MH, Flynn N (2002) Epidemiology and public health consequences of methamphetamine use in California's Central Valley. *Journal of Psychoactive Drugs* 34 (3): 313–319.

Grant KM, Kelley SS, Agrawal S, *et al.* (2007) Methamphetamine use in rural Midwesterners. *American Journal on Addictions* 16 (2): 79–84.

Gurnack AM, Paul W (1997) Factors related to perinatal substance abuse in a California county. *Perceptual and Motor Skills* 84 (3 Pt 2): 1403–1408.

Hall JA, Henggeler SW, Felice ME, *et al.* (1993) Adolescent substance use during pregnancy. *Journal of Pediatric Psychology* 18 (2): 265–271.

Herman-Stahl MA, Krebs CP, Kroutil LA, Heller DC (2006) Risk and protective factors for nonmedical use of prescription stimulants and methamphetamine among adolescents. *Journal of Adolescent Health* 39 (3): 374–380.

Herrell JM, Taylor JA, Gallagher C, Dawud-Noursi S (2000) A multisite study of the effectiveness of methamphetamine treatment: an initiative of the Center for Substance Abuse Treatment. *Journal of Psychoactive Drugs* 32 (2): 143–147.

Kosten TR, O'Connor PG (2003) Management of drug and alcohol withdrawal. *New England Journal of Medicine* 348 (18): 1786–1795.

Kresina TF, Normand J, Khalsa J, *et al.* (2004) Addressing the need for treatment paradigms for drug-abusing patients with multiple morbidities. *Clinical Infectious Diseases* 38 (Suppl. 5): S398–S401.

London ED, Simon SL, Berman SM, *et al.* (2004) Mood disturbances and regional cerebral metabolic abnormalities in recently abstinent methamphetamine abusers. *Archives of General Psychiatry* 61 (1): 73–84.

Luchansky B, Krupski A, Stark K (2007) Treatment response by primary drug of abuse: does methamphetamine make a difference? *Journal of Substance Abuse Treatment* 32 (1): 89–96.

McCaughan JA, Carlson RG, Falck RS, Siegal HA (2005) From "Candy Kids" to "Chemi-Kids": a typology of young adults who attend raves in the Midwestern United States. *Substance Use and Misuse* 40 (9–10): 1503–1523.

McGregor C, Srisurapanont M, Jittiwutikarn J, *et al.* (2005) The nature, time course and severity of methamphetamine withdrawal. *Addiction* 100 (9): 1320–1329.

McKetin R, McLaren J, Lubman DI, Hides L (2006) The prevalence of psychotic symptoms among methamphetamine users. *Addiction* 101 (10): 1473–1478.

Mecham N, Melini J (2002) Unintentional victims: development of a protocol for the care of children exposed to chemicals at methamphetamine laboratories. *Pediatric Emergency Care* 18 (4): 327–332.

Miller WR, Baca C, Compton WM, *et al.* (2006) Addressing substance abuse in health care settings. *Alcoholism: Clinical and Experimental Research* 30 (2): 292–302.

National Institutes of Health (2006) *NIDA InfoFacts: Methamphetamine.* Bethesda: National Institutes of Health: National Institute on Drug Abuse. www.nida.nih.gov/infofacts/methamphetamine.html.

Newton TF, Kalechstein AD, Duran S, Vansluis N, Ling W (2004) Methamphetamine abstinence syndrome: preliminary findings. *American Journal on Addictions* 13 (3): 248–255.

NTP-CERHR (2005) National Toxicology Program NTP-CERHR monograph on the potential human reproductive and developmental effects of amphetamines. *NTP CERHR Monograph* 16: vii–III1.

Perez-Reyes M, White WR, McDonald SA (1991) Clinical effects of daily methamphetamine administration. *Clinical Neuropharmacology* 14 (4): 352–358.

Rawson RA, Gonzales R, Marinelli-Casey P, Ang A (2007) Methamphetamine dependence: a closer look at treatment response and clinical characteristics associated with route of administration in outpatient treatment. *American Journal on Addictions* 16 (4): 291–299.

Reback CJ, Larkins S, Shoptaw S (2003) Methamphetamine abuse as a barrier to HIV medication adherence among gay and bisexual men. *AIDS Care* 15 (6): 775–785.

Roll JM (2007) Contingency management: an evidence-based component of methamphetamine use disorder treatments. *Addiction* 102 (Suppl. 1): 114–120.

Sexton RL, Carlson RG, Leukefeld CG, Booth BM (2006) Methamphetamine use and adverse consequences in the rural southern United States: an ethnographic overview. *Journal of Psychoactive Drugs* (Suppl. 3): 393–404.

Siegal HA, Draus PJ, Carlson RG, Falck RS, Wang J (2006) Perspectives on health among adult users of illicit stimulant drugs in rural Ohio. *Journal of Rural Health* 22 (2): 169–173.

Simons JS, Oliver MN, Gaher RM, Ebel G, Brummels P (2005) Methamphetamine and alcohol abuse and dependence symptoms: associations with affect lability and impulsivity in a rural treatment population. *Addictive Behaviors* 30 (7): 1370–1381.

Sommers I, Baskin D, Baskin-Sommers A (2006) Methamphetamine use among young adults: health and social consequences. *Addictive Behaviors* 31 (8): 1469–1476.

Springer AE, Peters RJ, Shegog R, White DL, Kelder SH (2007) Methamphetamine use and sexual risk behaviors in U.S. high school students: findings from a national risk behavior survey. *Prevention Science* 8 (2): 103–113.

Srisurapanont M, Sombatmai S, Boripuntakul T (2007) Brief intervention for students with methamphetamine use disorders: a randomized controlled trial. *American Journal on Addiction* 16 (2): 111–116.

Sulzer D, Sonders MS, Poulsen NW, Galli A (2005) Mechanisms of neurotransmitter release by amphetamines: a review. *Progress in Neurobiology* 75 (6): 406–433.

Sun AP (2007) Relapse among substance-abusing women: components and processes. *Substance Use & Misuse* 42 (1): 1–21.

Thorberg FA, Lyvers M (2006) Negative mood regulation (NMR) expectancies, mood, and affect intensity among clients in substance disorder treatment facilities. *Addictive Behaviors* 31 (5): 811–820.

Toumbourou JW, Stockwell T, Neighbors C, *et al.* (2007) Interventions to reduce harm associated with adolescent substance use. *Lancet* 369 (9570): 1391–1401.

US Department of Health and Human Services (2007) *Results from the 2006 National Survey on Drug Use and Health: National Findings*. Rockville: US Department of Health and Human Services Substance Abuse and Mental Health Services Administration Office of Applied Studies. http://www.oas.samhsa.gov/nsduh/2k6nsduh/2k6Results.pdf.

US Drug Enforcement Administration (2007) *National Drug Threat Assessment 2007: Methamphetamine*. US Department of Justice. www.usdoj.gov/dea/concern/18862/meth.htm.

Vik PW (2007) Methamphetamine use by incarcerated women: comorbid mood and anxiety problems. *Women's Health Issues* 17 (4): 256–263.

von MC, Brecht ML, Anglin MD (2002) Use ecology and drug use motivations of methamphetamine users admitted to substance abuse treatment facilities in Los Angeles: an emerging profile. *Journal of Addictive Diseases* 21 (1): 45–60.

Winslow BT, Voorhees KI, Pehl KA (2007) Methamphetamine abuse. *American Family Physician* 76 (8): 1169–1174.

Zule WA, Costenbader EC, Meyer WJ Jr, Wechsberg WM (2007) Methamphetamine use and risky sexual behaviors during heterosexual encounters. *Sexually Transmitted Diseases* 34 (9): 689–694.

Chapter 16

Public Health and Dual Diagnosis

Linda Bailey

Introduction

People accessing health care who present with a diagnosis of both mental illness and substance misuse pose a particular challenge for health services. This is because their condition may be further complicated by other factors associated with either their mental health diagnosis or their substance misuse, such as increased risk of in-patient admission, poor compliance with treatment, homelessness, violence, domestic violence, suicide, offending behaviour, or physical ill-health such as a blood-borne virus (BBV) or liver damage.

In examining the public health aspects of dual diagnosis, this chapter will focus on what is known about the epidemiology of dual diagnosis, the associated public health problems and implications and interventions available for dual diagnosis. It should also be remembered that while the term *dual diagnosis* implies the presence of two conditions, it is possible that a person presenting with both mental health problems and substance abuse may also be suffering from a number of other conditions. Further, much of the literature around dual diagnosis looks at the comorbidities of drug misuse and psychosis; however, other mental health conditions as well as misuse of alcohol must be considered.

Epidemiology

Ascertaining the size of the challenge is in itself difficult. Substance misuse is often not revealed to health care professionals because much of the substance misuse involves illegal drugs, although there are also issues with over-use of alcohol and self-medication with prescribed or 'over-the-counter' drugs.

In the general population with and without mental health problems, young adults have high exposure to illicit drugs – around half of the population aged 16–29 in England and Wales report having used an illicit drug, the majority using cannabis. There are specific issues related to the use of cannabis by young people in relation to dual diagnosis and strong suggestions of a causal link between cannabis use and psychosis. About 1.2 million people in England and Wales aged 16–24 report that they have also used an illicit psychoactive drug in the previous month (Marsden *et al.* 2004). Drug use is linked to social issues such as homelessness and social exclusion, and young people in the care system are more likely to misuse drugs than those not in care.

In terms of what is known about dual diagnosis, a study (Frisher *et al.* 2004) carried out in primary care using the national General Practice Research Database (GPRD) found that between 1993 and 1998 the comorbidity rate increased by about 10% each year, and co-morbid cases are becoming younger. This study excluded dependence on alcohol. Men were more likely to be diagnosed with substance misuse or dependence; however, women had a higher prevalence of licit dependence in the study. In both men and women prevalence of substance use declined with age.

A smaller study (Barnett *et al.* 2007) suggested that of those patients presenting to a service in the east of England with a first episode of psychosis, more than half were using cannabis and that substance use, including use of Class A drugs, was double that of the general population. The study also suggested that those who start taking drugs at a younger age delay seeking help for longer after their first psychotic episode.

Suicide and self harm are significant mental health issues with a strong link to both drug and alcohol misuse. A 25-year cohort study (Oyefeso *et al.* 1999) following up 69,880 notified addicts found that 82% of the 298 suicides recorded in the cohort were in men, the majority of whom were aged between 15 and 34. Forty-five percent of the suicides were by drug overdose. The risk of suicide for people who were notified addicts, when compared to the rest of the population, was four times higher for male addicts and 11 times higher for female addicts. A briefing paper from Alcohol Concern (2003) suggested that between 15% and 25% of suicides were related to alcoholism, and both substance misuse and alcohol misuse were associated with more repeat suicide attempts.

Prevalence studies among specific groups of the population have been carried out. People with a dual diagnosis are also more likely to have experience of being in prison because of the association with offending behaviour. In 1999 (Weild *et al.* 2000) 3930 prisoners from eight prisons in England and Wales completed a questionnaire on history of intravenous drug use (IVDU). Twenty-four percent of them reported a history of IVDU, and three quarters of those who admitted to having injected in prison (224/747) said they had shared injecting equipment in prison. One study looking at psychiatric morbidity in prisoners (Singleton *et al.* 1998) carried out by the Office of National Statistics found that 79% of male remand prisoners who were drug dependent also had two or more additional mental disorders.

Professionals dealing with female clients with a history of both mental illness and substance use need to be aware of the associations between dual diagnosis and domestic violence. An American study (McPherson *et al.* 2007) of 324 mothers with severe mental illness showed that 19% of the women had experienced domestic violence in the previous year and that women with a dual diagnosis were more likely than women without such a diagnosis to report experiencing domestic violence.

While little UK research is available, there are also thought to be variations in dual diagnosis patterns according to ethnicity. Miles *et al.* (2003) in a study carried out in South London found that clients who were alcohol dependent were significantly more likely to be of white European descent, while black Caribbean, black African and black British were more likely to be in the sub-group who misused cannabis. Ethnicity is also negatively associated with poorer access to health care services generally. However, it is easy to make erroneous generalisations based on ethnicity, and professionals working in the field of mental health should be alert to the existence of different cultural models of health and illness.

A major challenge for health care staff dealing with patients with a dual diagnosis is the link between drug and alcohol use and violent behaviour on in-patient wards. An audit carried out by the Healthcare Commission and the Royal College of Psychiatrists in 2007 (Healthcare Commission & Royal College of Psychiatrists 2007) found that 85% of nursing staff on acute psychiatric wards felt that their work was affected by incidents caused by clients' alcohol use. 'Problems can arise when service users deal or take drugs on the ward. This leads to increases in violence and aggression towards staff and between service users' (p. 63).

Causal relationship

While it is undeniable that there is a strong association between mental illness and substance misuse problems, studies are conflicting as to whether the association between mental illness and substance misuse is causal, i.e. does mental illness cause people to start taking drugs or does drug taking lead to mental illness?

In attempting to explain the comorbidity between mental illness and substance misuse, two suggestions feature more prominently in the literature:

- Anti-social personality disorder is a common factor leading to both.
- People who are predisposed to developing mental health problems are also likely to be sensitive to a number of risks for mental illness, substance abuse being one of the risks.

In epidemiological research, for an association to be deemed causal, certain criteria should be established. The nine criteria were described by Bradford-Hill (1965) and are as below:

- Strength – the strength of the association
- Consistency – whether the association is consistent across different studies by different people
- Specificity – whether the association is specific to certain populations at specific sites in the absence of alternative likely explanations
- Temporality – the effect should take place after the cause
- Biological gradient – the greater the exposure to the issue being investigated, then the greater the incidence of the effect
- Plausibility – whether the link between cause and effect makes sense
- Coherency – the association should not conflict with what is generally known about the natural history and biology of disease
- Experiment – whether there is experimental evidence available that will support the idea that the association is causal
- Analogy – whether there is another, similar association between two variables that would support the idea that a like made sense

Clearly, not all the above criteria need to apply for an association either way to be causal. In terms of substance misuse leading to mental health problems there have been a number of studies linking cannabis use to severe mental illness, and one review of five longitudinal studies (Smit *et al.* 2004) concluded that 'antecedent cannabis use appears to act as a risk factor in the onset of schizophrenia, especially in vulnerable people, but also in people without prior history'.

A further study in the *British Medical Journal* (BMJ) stated that exposure to cannabis use in adolescence and young adulthood increases the risk of psychotic symptoms later in life, but that this association is stronger for individuals with existing predisposition to psychosis (Henquet *et al.* 2005). There was also a dose–response relationship in that more frequent use of cannabis was linked to higher levels of risk.

Dual diagnosis and blood-borne infections

One of the more serious public health implications of intravenous drug misuse are BBVs such as Hepatitis B (HBV) and Hepatitis C (HCV) and HIV. Thus the population with dual diagnosis may be further affected by ill health due to a BBV. The BBV most commonly linked to intravenous drug misuse is HCV.

Hepatitis C

The prevalence of HCV is considerably higher in intravenous drug users (IVDUs) than in the general population, although there is little information about whether prevalence is higher in IVDUs with a dual diagnosis. It is certainly increased in IVDUs who are or have been homeless, which in itself is associated with mental illness. More than a third of IVDUs attending specialist services have evidence of infection, and some smaller studies have estimated this level to be between 50 and 80%.

When HCV prevalence is estimated by length of injecting, career one community survey (Department of Health 2001) showed HCV levels of

- less than 10% for those injecting for 2 years or less;
- about one-third for those injecting for between 6 and 8 years;
- over 75% for those injecting for 15 years or longer.

The prevalence of HCV in IVDUs in London has been found to be significantly higher than elsewhere in the United Kingdom. This could be due to under detection/diagnosis but may also be due to a real difference.

There are also suggestions that HCV may be spread between drug users snorting or sniffing drugs through sharing banknotes, so the disease may not be confined to those using drugs intravenously.

Hepatitis B

Overall about one in five IVDUs have had HBV infection (Health Protection Agency 2007). In 2003 injecting drug use was the main risk associated with HBV infection, accounting for 34% of individuals with a known risk factor in England, and 27% in Wales. Despite the availability of an effective vaccine for HBV, prevalence has continued to increase in IVDUs.

Human immunodeficiency virus

The prevalence of HIV infection among IVDUs in England and Wales has continued to rise since the virus was first identified. Overall, around one in 75 IVDUs now have HIV infection, which is still low, compared to many other countries. The prevalence is elevated among current IVDUs in London with around 1 in 20 HIV-infected. Again this is not specific to those drug users with dual diagnosis, but applicable to all drug users.

Treatment for BBV

There is currently no vaccine available to prevent the spread of HCV or HIV; however, a vaccine exists that offers protection against HBV. Treatment for HCV and HBV now exists, which will clear the viruses in 40–50% of those infected. However, advice varies as to whether those people who are HCV/HBV positive but still using drugs should be offered the antiviral treatment available. There is treatment which will address symptoms of HIV and slow the progress of HIV disease but there is no treatment which will clear the HIV virus. There is some evidence to support the use of post-exposure prophylaxis in people who have been exposed to HIV.

The National Institute for Clinical Excellence (NICE) recommends (NICE 2004) pegylated interferon alfa and ribavirin for the treatment of HCV. However, about half of the people treated suffer side effects from the treatment, such as fatigue, headaches, temperature, myalgia, insomnia and nausea. About a quarter suffer hair loss, arthralgia, rigors, irritability, pruritus, depression and dermatitis. These side effects mean that there are significant problems of patients not complying with or completing treatment. NICE estimated treatment dropout rates of 7–14%, and while this may be higher in those people still using drugs, NICE recommends that they should still be offered treatment.

Other co-infections

Apart from being at a greatly increased risk of developing a BBV, people using intravenous drugs are also at increased risk from other serious infections, usually from sharing injecting kit, but also linked to the actual substance being injected. These infections include staphylococcal and streptococcal infections, and clostridial infections such as wound botulism (*Clostridium botulinum*) and tetanus (*Clostridium tetani*). There is also an increased risk of sexually transmitted infections among people who misuse drugs, as they are more likely to engage in unprotected sexual intercourse. This is more likely in people using intravenous drugs than in those using cannabis.

Prevention and intervention

Prevention is traditionally seen as being one of the three strands of health promotion, the others being health education and health protection. Prevention is usually classified under three subheadings (Donaldson & Donaldson 2000):

- *Primary prevention:* This approach is aimed at preventing the onset or acquisition of disease. It includes the giving of information, although this may be utilised at the secondary and tertiary stages too. It also includes immunisation and environmental changes.
- *Secondary prevention:* This is aimed at preventing the progress of a disease once it is established, and includes screening, early diagnosis and timely, effective treatment.

- *Tertiary prevention:* This is the approach taken with people who have an existing disease or condition, such as the provision of rehabilitation and the promotion of independent living.

In the context of preventive strategies in dual diagnosis with those who use intravenous drugs, the first two are particularly important. Preventative programmes which have been found to be effective (Canning *et al.* 2003) in young people are programmes which modify attitudes and normative beliefs. Examples of primary prevention would include provision of HBV vaccine, needle exchange programmes (NEP), making condoms available, and information giving. However, offering substitute treatment to drug users to enable them to stop using intravenous drugs may also be considered primary prevention. Secondary prevention would include strategies such as screening for disease and prompt treatment to those infected. It may also include interventions such as offering HIV post-exposure prophylaxis where there has been needle sharing and ensuring that treatment and care continued in a population which is often highly mobile. While there are needle exchanges available in the United Kingdom, a BMJ article (Judd *et al.* 2005) suggested that they provided a clean needle to users on average once every 2 days, which may not be frequent enough to prevent transmission of all BBVs, given that the prevalence of BBVs is continuing to rise.

Interventions for dual diagnosis should be based on evidence of effectiveness. There are a number of models available, such as the Comprehensive, Continuous, Integrated System of Care (CCISC) model from United States described by Kenneth Minkoff (2005) which calls for a system-wide approach using an integrated philosophy of care based on the use of a common language of care between service providers, whether they are primarily a mental health or a substance misuse service.

This and other successful approaches use a 'stages of change' model which encompasses a number of phases in the treatment cycle – acute stabilisation, motivational enhancement, active treatment, relapse prevention, and rehabilitation and recovery. In this approach, interventions are not only specific to the diagnosis, but they are also specific to the person's stage of change and recovery.

The 'Stages of Change' model was originally developed in the late 1970s by Prochaska and DiClemente (1994), and is a useful model used in health promotion and public health when looking at changing behaviour in relation to addictions, be that addiction to nicotine, food, alcohol or drugs. The model is cyclical and the stages of change they described are given below:

- *Pre-contemplation:* When an individual has not yet identified that they have a behaviour in need of change. Until this acknowledgement occurs within an individual, any attempts to impose behaviour change or support them will probably fail.

- *Contemplation:* The person has identified that there is a problem but may not be ready or sure of wanting to make the necessary changes.
- *Preparation:* The need to change has been identified and the individual makes plans as to how to address the problem. They will identify the support they need and take actions such as ensuring that support is there and setting a date on which they will start to make changes.
- *Change:* The changes in behaviour are implemented.
- *Maintenance:* Maintaining the behaviour change.
- *Relapse:* This may occur at any stage of the model, and should be seen as part of the cycle rather than a failure.

Where prevention has not worked, intervention is necessary. However, given that social exclusion and homelessness are strongly associated with illicit drug use, effective interventions are difficult to deliver, and users find it even more difficult to adhere to treatment programmes. A key part of any successful treatment programme should therefore include addressing some of the social issues by providing clients with stable accommodation and an income.

Successful treatment of dual diagnosis in the United Kingdom may be hindered by the fact that historically different teams of professionals dealt with each aspect of the disorder, with drug and alcohol teams focusing on the substance misuse and others focusing on the mental health problem. And rather than a holistic approach being taken, the conditions were often dealt with by different professionals at different times, with the client themselves often being expected to provide liaison and coordination between the different teams. In 2002, the Department of Health published a dual diagnosis good practice guide calling for mainstreaming and greater integration of services (Department of Health 2002). Models of care have also been developed nationally.

There may be different aims for intervention, especially if abstinence is an unrealistic aspiration for some clients. One focus for intervention is harm reduction. Rather than trying to assist clients to become free of their addiction, interventions may be aimed at helping them manage their addiction so that the risks are greatly reduced.

Conclusion

Co-occurring mental health and substance misuse problems are highly prevalent today and the prevalence appears to be increasing. This could be a genuine increase; it could also be due to more robust diagnosis, or it could be due to the increasing medicalisation of social conditions. More research into the epidemiology is needed to give greater understanding of the conditions involved, and to plan appropriate services. Specifically, more large-scale cohort and longitudinal studies will give insight into the issues.

However, clients with a dual diagnosis are a heterogeneous group, and not all the issues identified will apply to everyone with a dual diagnosis, nor will their service needs be the same. Historically in UK health care, a medical approach has been used to address mental health problems, and a psychosocial approach has been taken with people with substance abuse problems. Services now are changing slowly to take a more holistic approach to treating people with dual diagnosis. But there is a lack of robust research into effective interventions in dual diagnosis and more work is needed in this area.

References

Alcohol Concern (2003) *Mental Health & Alcohol Misuse Project: Briefing 5 – Suicide and Alcohol Misuse.* London: Alcohol Concern.

Barnett JH, Werners U, Secher SM, *et al.* (2007) Substance use in a population-based clinic sample of people with first-episode psychosis. *British Journal of Psychiatry* 190: S15–S20.

Bradford-Hill A (1965) The Environment and disease: association or causation? Presidential address to the section of Occupational Medicine of the Royal Society of Medicine, London.

Canning U, Millward L, Raj T (2003) *Drug Use Prevention: A Review of Reviews. Evidence Briefing Summary.* London: Heath Development Agency.

Department of Health (2001) *Hepatitis C – Guidance for Those Working With Drug Users.* London: Department of Health pp. 4–5.

Department of Health (2002) *Mental Health Policy Implementation Guide: Dual Diagnosis Good Practice Guidance.* London: Department of Health.

Donaldson LJ, Donaldson RJ (2000) *Essential Public Health*, 2nd Edition. Plymouth: Petroc Press.

Frisher M, Collins J, Millson D, Crome I, Croft P (2004) Prevalence of comorbid psychiatric illness and substance misuse in primary care in England and Wales. *Journal of Epidemiology & Community Health* 58: 1036–1041.

Healthcare Commission & Royal College of Psychiatrists (2007) *The Healthcare Commission National Audit of Violence 2006–7: Final Report – Working Age Adult Services.* London: Royal College of Psychiatrists.

Health Protection Agency (2007) *Shooting up. Infections among Injecting Drug Users in the United Kingdom 2006: An Update in October 2007.* London: Health Protection Agency.

Henquet C, Krabbendam L, Spauwen J, *et al.* (2005) Prospective cohort study of cannabis use, predisposition for psychosis, and psychotic symptoms in young people. *British Medical Journal* 330: 11–17.

Judd A, Hickman M, Jones S, *et al.* (2005) Incidence of hepatitis C virus and HIV among new injecting drug users in London: prospective cohort study. *British Medical Journal* 330: 24–25.

Marsden J, Strang J, Lavoie D, Abdulrahim D, Hickman M, Scott S (2004) Healthcare needs assessment: the epidemiologically based needs assessment reviews – drug misuse Accessed 12/2/08. http://www.hcna.bham.ac.uk/chapters.shtml.

McPherson MD, Delva J, Cranford JA (2007) A longitudinal investigation of intimate partner violence among mothers with mental illness. *Psychiatric Services* 58 (5): 675–680.

Miles H, Johnson S, Amponsah-Afuwape S, *et al.* (2003) Characteristics of subgroups of individuals with psychotic illness and a comorbid substance use disorder by substance of choice. *Psychiatric Services* 54: 554–564.

Minkoff K (2005) The Comprehensive, Continuous, Integrated System of Care (CCISC) model. www.kenminkoff.com/ccisc.html.

National Institute for Clinical Excellence (2004) *Technology Appraisal Guidance 75: Interferon Alfa (Pegylated and Non-pegylated) and Ribavirin for the Treatment for Chronic Hepatitis C*. London: NICE.

Oyefeso A, Ghodse H, Clancy C, Corkery J (1999) Suicide among drug addicts in the UK. *British Journal of Psychiatry* 175: 277–282.

Prochaska JO, DiClemente CC (1994) *The Transtheoretical Approach: Crossing Traditional Boundaries of Therapy*. Malabar (Florida): Krieger Publishing.

Singleton N, Meltzer H, Gatward R, Coid J, Deasy D (1998) *Psychiatric Morbidity among Prisoners in England and Wales: Summary*. London: The Stationery Office.

Smit F, Bolier L, Cuijpers P (2004) Cannabis use and the risk of later schizophrenia: a review. *Addiction* 99: 425–430.

Weild AR, Gill ON, Bennett D, Livingstone SJ, Parry JV, Curran L (2000) Prevalence of HIV, hepatitis B, and hepatitis C antibodies in prisoners in England and Wales: a national survey *Communicable Disease & Public Health* 3: 121–126.

Chapter 17

Comorbidity or Complexity: A Primary Care Perspective on Dual Diagnosis

John Budd

Introduction

In the National Health Service (NHS) the majority of health care is provided in primary care and this is generally estimated to be somewhere in the region of 90% of all patient contacts. In the case of dual diagnosis, very little is known of what care is actually provided in the primary care setting, although there is evidence that primary care is playing an increasingly significant role (Frisher *et al.* 2004).

In the United Kingdom, the term primary care refers to the health care services provided by community-based health professionals working in general practice clinics, along with allied services. The general practitioners (GPs), who commonly own these clinics, are independent contractors working for the NHS and are often seen as the fulcrum of the primary care service. GPs are primary care physicians with a wide general medical training. Other health care professionals who routinely work within the primary care team include practice nurses, health visitors and district nurses (community nurses), along with community midwives. GPs and primary care nurses are for most people the first point of contact with the NHS. This service is state funded, free at the point of delivery and fulfils a gatekeeping role for the NHS. It offers care and treatment, but also refers patients on to appropriate specialist services for investigations or treatments that are outwith the scope of the generalist care provided in primary care.

This is very much a medical model of primary care and quite different from the concept of primary care as expressed by the World Health Organization through such documents as the Alma Ata declaration (WHO 1978). Here, a more social model of primary health care is articulated that is more participatory, more politicised and has a strong ethos of community development.

Elsewhere in this volume, dual diagnosis has been defined as the co-occurrence of severe mental illness along with substance misuse, meaning either drug or alcohol problems or both. However, from a primary care perspective, the definition could be meaningfully expanded to encompass the idea of complexity. This is of particular relevance given that the relationship between mental health disorders and substance misuse is in itself a complex one and that often a distinction between the primary and secondary diagnoses cannot easily be made. It could also be argued that, by definition, anyone using substances in a heavily dependent way has significant mental health problems.

The Cartesian philosophical concept of the mind–body divide underlies this diagnostic duality, with the representation of these problems as two discrete entities having more to do with the division and design of services than any meaningful clinical reality. The recognition of the centrality of complexity would actually offer the potential for a more flexible and integrated service response, which should be core to meeting the needs of this group of patients.

A more functional definition would include mental health and substance misuse problems, along with the social and physical problems that are very much within the remit of the primary care clinician. Therefore, in this chapter, the term comorbidity will be used to refer to patients suffering from a complexity of issues of which mental health and substance misuse problems are a part. The case study below gives an example of the complexity of problems that can be encountered and potentially addressed in primary care, when working in collaboration with other appropriate services. It also gives an idea of the pragmatic risk management approach that is characteristic of the health care provided in general practice and it highlights the failings of having fragmented and perhaps rigid specialist services.

CASE STUDY 1

PB is a 28-year-old white male. He spent several years in care as a child due to parental alcohol problems. He has been diagnosed with borderline personality disorder, schizophrenia and has a long history of opiate dependence. He has been in and out of touch with mental health and substance misuse services over many years, with periods of homelessness. The only continuity in his health care has been provided by his GP, who has maintained him on methadone treatment and an antipsychotic, chlorpromazine, for his psychiatric disorder.

Over recent months there has been a deterioration in his mental health, with agitation and persecutory ideation following his being a victim of a violent assault. This led to a relapse into injecting heroin and a further episode of homelessness.

PB was referred to the community mental health team but did not engage with them. The GP then linked him in with a local non-statutory support agency that helped PB access emergency accommodation. The GP also increased his methadone dose and increased his chlorpromazine.

His agitation started to improve, but shortly after this, he became yellow with jaundice and developed severe sweats and blackouts. He refused hospital admission and as his mental health was improving, he was not detainable. Serological blood tests confirmed an acute hepatitis C infection. Over subsequent weeks, the sweats and blackouts were becoming increasingly problematic and could have been due to the chlorpromazine or the methadone or a drug interaction between them. An ECG and cardiac monitoring were arranged, but PB kept failing to attend for these investigations.

The GP decided that since PB's social situation was stabilising it would be safe to reduce his chlorpromazine. PB tolerated this well and the sweats and blackouts resolved. He is now in settled accommodation, is stable on methadone treatment and off illicit drugs and has been enlisted in a work-training programme by the non-statutory agency. He continues to see his GP every 2 weeks and has been referred to the local hospital hepatitis C service.

Policy framework

The recently published new UK national guidelines on the management of drug use have underlined the central place of general practice in the management of substance misuse (DH 2007). With regard to dual diagnosis, although mainstream mental health services have been identified as the best place for the treatment of co-morbid patients, the national guidelines recognise general practice as having a key role to play (DH 2002). Both these and the more recent Scottish 'Closing the Gaps' report describe the role of the GP in identification, assessment, appropriate referral, and provision of care. The English document specifically defines this provision of care in terms of physical health; however, the Scottish report suggests a wider role for primary care (Scottish Government 2007).

Primary care is seen to fit into a tiered structure of services as advocated by the National Treatment Agency (NTA), with general practice as a tier one service, focusing on patients with less specialised needs. Patients with more complex needs are to be referred on up the tiers to a more specialised service as appropriate. For this design to function, close working links between the tiers are essential, to facilitate easy patient movement through the service structure according to their needs. In this context, the national guidance recommends a collaborative approach to the management of patients with co-morbid mental health and substance misuse disorders (NTA 2002).

Epidemiology

The epidemiology of dual diagnosis has been discussed elsewhere in this text, so will only be touched on here; however, the data as it pertains to primary care will be discussed in more detail. In general, substance misuse is usual, rather than exceptional, among those with severe mental illness. Among those with a substance misuse problem, mental health disorders are common, reported as 30% in alcohol dependence and 45% in drug dependence (Farrell *et al.* 2001).

The high prevalence rates for comorbidity in these patient groups have been confirmed by studies such as the COSMIC study with even higher rates found for mental illness in both alcohol and drug treatment groups (Weaver *et al.* 2002). Surveys have also confirmed this practice, with particularly high prevalence of comorbidity in certain population groups, such as those in psychiatric patients in institutional care and among those who experience homelessness (Farrell *et al.* 1998).

With rising prevalence figures, it is of no surprise that the rate of comorbidity of psychiatric illness and substance misuse in primary care is also rising. A study using the general practice research database found a 62% increase in prevalence among co-morbid patients being cared for in primary care over a 5-year study period to 1998. They concluded that general practice is playing an increasingly important role in the management of comorbidity. Indeed, they extrapolated their findings to estimate that the average general practice will care for 14 chronic co-morbid patients in 2006, up 100% from seven patients in 1998 (Frisher *et al.* 2004). Interestingly, a further study using this database investigated the nature of the relationship between substance misuse and mental illness in primary care in the United Kingdom (Frisher *et al.* 2005). It concluded that the rise in comorbidity is not attributable to increasing substance misuse; however, a significant amount of substance misuse may be attributable to psychiatric illness. Once again, it is the high rate of comorbidity in primary care that is significant.

One area that is often overlooked is the relationship of both substance misuse and mental illness with deprivation. Severe mental illness shows a close correlation with deprivation (McLaren & Bain 1998), as do more minor mental illnesses, such as anxiety and depression, to a lesser degree (Stirling *et al.* 2001). In the most disadvantaged groups, such as those experiencing homelessness, rates of personality disorder have been reported to be as high as 70% (Burley *et al.* 2002). In a primary care population with substance misuse problems, it is the high prevalence of these mild and moderate mental health disorders that make up the majority of the co-morbid patients (Strathdee *et al.* 2002).

In terms of drug dependency, there is again a close correlation with deprivation. With alcohol, the picture is more complicated; however, the important fact is that the morbidity and mortality of harmful and dependent alcohol use is experienced disproportionately in deprived communities. Indeed, the mortality associated with alcohol in deprived groups is comparable to their mortality risk for coronary heart disease with a sevenfold increase in alcohol-related mortality in the most deprived categories compared to the most affluent (Scottish Executive 2002).

When looking at co-morbid mental health and substance misuse disorders in terms of deprivation, there is a lack of research into combined substance misuse and psychiatric illness; however, there is research in other areas showing that the prevalence of comorbidities rises with increasing poverty and deprivation (Macleod *et al.* 2004). This clustering of comorbidity in disadvantaged groups and communities is an important factor in the health inequalities experienced by these groups. As the NHS seeks to respond to the government's health inequalities agenda, this should have a significant impact on resource allocation and service development (Mercer & Watt 2007).

Key features of general practice care

Central to general practice is a long-term, patient-centred, therapeutic relationship. This is not established on the basis of a particular diagnosis, but rather starts from where the patient is and seeks to address their health needs in a broad, holistic way that includes health promotion, prevention and treatment. This relationship is often built up slowly, even over years, with the principle of 'cradle to the grave' care still an important foundation for general practice care.

General practice is the only service that can offer this life-long care. In fact, since the advent of care in the community, there are very few long-term health services, with the exception of the few remaining long-term residential psychiatric institutions and long-term psychotherapy. It is this core feature of general practice that makes it the ideal service setting for the management and care of patients with chronic disease. General practice does not seek to discharge patients, but rather sees successful outcomes in terms of maintaining patient engagement and compliance with treatment.

Drake *et al.* (1993), using an evidence-based approach, have identified nine key features for a successful service for the treatment of those with co-morbid substance misuse and mental health disorders. One of these features is this long-term approach to the management of chronic and relapsing conditions. It is important to recognise that many patients with co-morbid substance misuse and psychiatric illness – particularly those with more severe mental illness – are likely to benefit from long-term service engagement, with easy and immediate access as may be needed during times of crises and relapse.

In general practice, patients are seen in their social settings within their homes, families and communities, and relationships are built across generations, often giving a very vivid family history. General practice is also able to offer assertive outreach, with GPs and community nurses offering home visiting as a core part of their work both for acute care and also for chronic disease management and follow-up.

With this move towards chronic disease management in general practice, the care offered has become increasingly shared across the primary care team. This integrated team approach has brought to bear a wide range of clinical skills, involving GPs, practice nurses, nurse practitioners, district nurses and health visitors. This has allowed for increasing health promotion and prevention interventions, such as brief interventions being given by practice and community nurses. Another key feature identified in the approach of general practice to the management of substance misuse is that of flexibility, which is again of particular importance in the care of co-morbid patients (DH 2002). In this setting, the co-morbid patient, if engaged and held in contact, has the opportunity to experience a holistic form of care that meets most of the key features of Drake *et al.* (1993) for a successful service.

Physical health care

Physical health care is a crucial part of the holistic care for patients who have co-morbid mental health and substance misuse disorders. This can be all too easily overlooked when dealing with hard-to-engage patients who suffer with low self-esteem and who often seem indifferent to the state of their physical health.

In this patient group, there is a high prevalence of physical comorbidities, which may be as a consequence of the substance misuse or associated with the mental health disorder or its treatment. Those with severe mental illness are at increased risk for HIV, hepatitis B, hepatitis C and sexually transmitted disease (Rosenberg *et al.* 2001). Schizophrenia, depression and substance misuse disorders are associated with an increased risk of cardiovascular disease and other chronic diseases, yet these patients face significant barriers in accessing medical services and treatment, which results in premature death for many (DRC 2006). This increased risk may be due to an increase in all the modifiable risk behaviours, including smoking, high alcohol intake, poor diet, lack of exercise and obesity (Davidson *et al.* 2001), and in the case of schizophrenia and depression, pharmacotherapy can add to the metabolic changes causing further increased risk.

The cardiotoxic effects of many substances such as alcohol and stimulants are well recognised. Alcohol is further associated with a wide range of ill-health effects from gastro-intestinal, liver and pancreatic disease, to neurological damage such as cognitive impairment, dementia and increased risk of strokes. It is also now well recognised that heavy and prolonged benzodiazepine use is associated with permanent cognitive impairment. Co-morbid mental health and substance misuse patients are at increased risk of suicide (Bakken & Valgum 2007), with older male injecting drug users being at particular risk of overdose and death (Bird *et al.* 2003).

Substance misusers are not only at risk for the toxic effects of the substance used, but also for infectious diseases either through high-risk sexual behaviour (Butterfield *et al.* 2003) or through injecting. For stimulant users, benzodiazepine users and injecting drug users this includes HepA, HepB, HepC and HIV (HPA 2006). Injecting drug users are at risk of heart valve damage with sub-acute bacterial endocarditis, soft tissue infections and vascular damage that can lead to deep vein thrombosis and pulmonary embolus.

Thus the range of potential physical health problems that are added to the complexity of co-morbid patients can be seen. Primary care has the potential to address these health care needs, particularly through offering effective educational, clinical and harm-reducing interventions. This is an important part of the overall comprehensive care needed by co-morbid patients and it can enhance the therapeutic relationship, as well as contribute to improved mental health.

Mental health and substance misuse care

The extent to which co-morbid patients fall between services is a very real problem, as most primary care clinicians are only too aware. Patients with substance misuse problems managed in the community often have mental health problems that do not meet the criteria for referral to the mental health services (Strathdee *et al.* 2002) and similarly patients in community treatment for serious mental illness will frequently have a substance misuse problem that does not easily fit into an opiate-orientated substance misuse service (Weaver *et al.* 2003). If the serious mental illness is currently reasonably stable, again the patient may not be actively involved with mental health services. It is in this context that a more functional definition of comorbidity would be of particular relevance.

The stigma and negative attitudes found among some mental health workers towards substance misusers has been well documented and is another reason that the co-morbid patient might no longer be engaged with mental health services (Coombes & Wratten 2007). Furthermore, mental health and substance misuse services are often separate, with different philosophical approaches. This raises further barriers to effective engagement, leading many co-morbid patients to be reliant on primary care for all their ongoing care.

In this context, it is clear that a collaborative approach between services would offer the greatest potential to improve care. Perhaps, in an American setting, where there is a poorly developed primary care service, a specialist-integrated service may be optimum (Abou-Saleh 2007); however, in the United Kingdom this is not the case. What are needed from the primary care perspective are clearly defined care pathways, with good access to and rapid response from specialist services when required. For the more complex and difficult to manage co-morbid patients, ongoing specialist support will be needed and the main role for the GP may well be that of care coordinator, affording continuity of care, keeping patients engaged in treatment and liaising with social care (Gerada 2005).

Limitations and potential in primary care

Despite GPs having been encouraged for several years to take on the management of substance misuse, there are still only about one-third of GPs who are actively involved in prescribing substitute medication for drug users (NTA 2007). This suggests that there remains a significant untapped service capacity. Alternatively, this could also be interpreted as another example of the negative attitude of health workers to this patient group. However, it is often found that when offered relevant training and when they feel clinically supported by specialist colleagues, GPs are willing to undertake this work.

One area of collaborative working where general practice is often poor is working in partnership with local non-statutory services. This failure to link in with local substance misuse or mental health agencies, which can offer a psychosocial or key working support, has been identified as a significant factor in limiting patient's rehabilitation potential (SACDM 2007). This could also be seen as an inherent failing in the medical model of primary care and so an important area that needs to be addressed. For this to happen, GPs need to be confident of the quality and professional ethos of the non-statutory work force. In order to establish this, local experience in our service has shown there is no substitute for establishing face to face relationships with workers in other sectors for generating the trust and understanding needed for genuine partnership working.

The negative attitudes prevalent among some mental health workers towards substance misusing patients have already been identified as a potential barrier to care. These attitudes are also found among the primary care work force and pose a significant challenge (Peckover & Chidlaw 2007). These attitudes need to be actively addressed through training at both pre- and post-qualification levels for all primary care workers, in order to change this culture.

Training is key to addressing the untapped potential in primary care. The current national Royal College of General Practitioners (RCGP) drug misuse training programme for GPs and other primary care workers is a welcome and much-needed development. However, much more is needed at both the undergraduate and postgraduate levels to not only equip doctors and nurses with the necessary clinical skills, but more importantly to foster the non-judgmental attitude that can allow the worker to see the potential in working with patients to address their problems of addiction. This is essential to encourage the positive attitude – identified as a key service feature by Drake *et al.* (1993) – to these challenging, but often rewarding, patients.

The new General Medical Service contract for general practice has inhibited the development of care for substance misusing and co-morbid patients, but it has within it the seeds for positive change. Neither the management of alcohol problems nor drug problems falls within the core contract, but there is a provision made to offer a service for both as 'enhanced services'. The potential for the development of either local or national enhanced services that both recognise and provide for the care needs of this patient group is there. However, this depends on commissioners prioritising and funding these services and general practices being willing to opt in.

Conclusion

Primary care has a pivotal and often unrecognised role to play in the provision of care for this marginalised and vulnerable patient group. It is ideally suited to work in a collaborative way with more specialised services to provide the holistic health care required to meet their complex and multiple needs. To optimise this potential, it is vital that primary care is involved in both the planning and coordination of local services and that the contractual and training needs of primary care are addressed.

References

Abou-Saleh M (2007) Dual diagnosis: management in a psychosocial context. In: Day E (ed). *Clinical Topics in Addiction*. London: The Royal College of Psychiatrists.

Bakken K, Vaglum P (2007) Predictors of suicide attempters in substance dependent patients: a six year prospective follow-up. *Clinical Practice and Epidemiology in Mental Health* 3: 20.

Bird S, Hutchison S, Goldberg D (2003) Drug-related deaths by region, sex and age group per 100 injecting drug users in Scotland, 2000-01. *The Lancet* 362: 941–944.

Burley A, Worthington H, Murphy T (2002) Homelessness and personality disorder. Unpublished research. Edinburgh Homeless Practice.

Butterfield M, Bosworth H, Meador K, *et al.* (2003) Gender differences in hepatitis C infection and risks among persons with severe mental illnes. *Psychiatric Services* 54: 848–853.

Coombes L, Wratten A (2007) The lived experience of community mental health nurses working with people who have dual diagnosis: a phenomenological study. *Journal of Psychiatric and Mental Health Nursing* 14: 382–392.

Davidson S, Judd F, Jolley D, *et al.* (2001) Cardiovascular risk factors for people with mental illness. *Australian and New Zealand Journal of Psychiatry* 35: 192–202.

Department of Health (2002) *Mental Health Policy Implementation Guide: Dual Diagnosis Good Practice Guide*. London: Department of Health.

Department of Health (England) and the Developed Administrations (2007) *Drug Misuse and Dependence: UK Guidelines on Clinical Management*. London: Department of Health (England), the Scottish Government, Welsh Assembly Government and Northern Ireland Executive.

Disability Rights Commission (2006) *Equal Treatment: Closing the Gap – A Formal Investigation into Physical Health Inequalities Experienced by People with Learning Disabilities and or Mental Health Problems*. London: DRC.

Drake R, Bartel S, Teague G, *et al.* (1993) Treatment of substance abuse in severely mentally ill patients. *The Journal of Nervous and Mental Disease* 181: 606–611.

Farrell M, Howes S, Bebbington P, *et al.* (2001) Nicotine, alcohol and drug dependence and psychiatric co-morbidity. Results of a national household survey. *British Journal of Psychiatry* 179: 432–437.

Farrell M, Howes S, Taylor C, *et al.* (1998) Substance misuse and psychiatric comorbidity. An overview of the OPCS national psychiatric morbidity survey. *Addictive Behaviours* 23: 909–918.

Frisher M, Collins J, Millson D, *et al.* (2004) Prevalence of comorbid psychiatric illness and substance misuse in primary care in England and Wales. *Journal of Epidemiology and Community Health* 58: 1036–1041.

Frisher M, Crome I, Macleod J, *et al.* (2005) Substance misuse and psychiatric illness: prospective observational study using the general practice research database. *Journal of Epidemiology and Community Health* 59: 847–850.

Gerada C (2005) Drug misuse and co-morbid illness: 'dual diagnosis'. In: Gerada C (ed). *RCGP Guide to the Management of Substance Misuse in Primary Care*. London: Royal College of General Practitioners.

Health Protection Agency (2006) *Shooting Up: Infections among Injecting Drug Users in the United Kingdom. An Update: October 2007*. London: HPA.

Macleod U, Mitchell E, Black M, Spence G (2004) Comorbidity and socioeconomic deprivation: an observation study of the prevalence of comorbidity in general practice. *The European Journal of General Practice* 10: 24–26.

McLaren G, Bain M (1998) *Deprivation and Health in Scotland. Insights from NHS Data*. Edinburgh: ISD Scotland Publications.

Mercer S, Watt G (2007) The Inverse Care Law: Clinical primary care encounters in deprived and affluent areas of Scotland. *Annals of Family Medicine* 5: 503–510.

National Treatment Agency for Substance Misuse (2002) *Models of Care for the Treatment of Drug Misuse.* London: NTA.

National Treatment Agency (2007) *The NTA's 2006 National Prescribing Audit: An Assessment of Prescribing Practices for Opioid Substitution Treatment in England, 2004–2005.* London: NTA.

Peckover S, Chidlaw R (2007) Too frightened to care? Accounts by district nurses working with clients who misuse substances. *Health and Social Care in the Community* 15: 238–245.

Rosenberg S, Goodman L, Oscher F, *et al.* (2001) Prevalence of HIV, hepatitis B and hepatitis C in people with severe mental illness. *American Journal of Public Health* 91: 31–37.

SACDM Methadone Project Group (2007) *Reducing Harm and Promoting Recovery: a Report on Methadone Treatment for Substance Misuse in Scotland.* Edinburgh: Scottish Advisory Council on Drug Misuse.

Scottish Executive (2002) *Plan for Action on Alcohol Problems.* Edinburgh: Scottish Executive.

Scottish Government (2007) *Mental Health in Scotland. Closing the Gaps – Making a Difference. Commitment 13.* Edinburgh: Scottish Government.

Stirling AM, Wilson P, McConnachie A (2001) Deprivation, psychological distress and consultation length general practice. *The British Journal of General Practice* 467: 456–460.

Strathdee G, Manning V, Best D, *et al.* (2002) *Dual Diagnosis in a Primary Care Group: A Step-by-Step Epidemiological Needs Assessments and Design of a Training and Service Response Model.* Report commissioned by Department of Health. Research Summary, 2004. London: NTA.

Weaver T, Charles V, Madden P, Renton P (2002) *Co-morbidity of Substance Misuse and Mental Illness Collaborative Study (COSMIC). A Study of the Prevalence and Management of Co-morbidity amongst Adult Substance Misuse and Mental Health Treatment Populations.* Research Summary, 2004. London: NTA.

Weaver T, Madden P, Charles V, *et al.* (2003) Comorbidity of substance misuse and mental illness in community mental health and substance misuse services. *The British Journal of Psychiatry* 183: 304–313.

WHO (1978) *Primary Health Care. Report on the International Conference on PHC at Alma Ata.* Geneva: WHO.

Part 3

International Perspectives, Policy and Development

Chapter 18

Dual Diagnosis – North America

Theodora Sirota and Kathleen Leo

Introduction

This chapter gives an overview of dual diagnosis in the United States. Prevalence, historical perspectives, socio-cultural and public policy issues, and approaches to treatment and research are reviewed and discussed. Treatment models in current use are described and existing problems and issues within the field are highlighted.

Prevalence

Co-occurring mental illness and substance use disorders constitute a serious public health problem in the United States, impacting our economy, workforce, welfare and educational and justice systems (IOM 2005). Data indicate that between 7 and 10 million individuals in the United States have co-occurring psychiatric illness and substance use disorders (President's New Freedom Commission on Mental Health 2003). SAMHSA (2004) reported that between 15 and 43% of the time, mental illnesses and substance use disorders are co-occurring. Gallagher *et al.* (2006) estimated that up to 51% of those with lifetime mental illness also suffer from lifetime substance abuse disorders. The National Comorbidity Study (Kessler *et al.* 1994) indicated that an estimated 78% of men and 86% of women who were alcohol dependent met the criteria for a lifetime diagnosis of another psychiatric disorder, including drug dependence. Data from the study also indicated that about 42.7% of adults aged 15–54 who had a substance disorder also had a mental illness and 14.7% of those with a mental illness had a co-occurring substance disorder (Kessler *et al.* 1994).

It is recognised that substance use disorders co-occur with a variety of mental illnesses such as depression, bipolar disorder, and anxiety disorders including post-traumatic stress disorder (PTSD) (IOM 2005). Grant *et al.* (2004) reported that approximately 20% of persons with substance use disorders have co-occurring anxiety or mood disorders. They also found that 60.3% of persons seeking help for a drug use disorder met the criteria for a mood disorder, 42.6% had anxiety disorders, and 55.2% had a co-morbid alcohol use disorder.

Especially high rates of co-occurring psychiatric and substance use disorders are seen in vulnerable populations in the United States. Gonzalez and Rosenheck (2002) reported that 43% of serious and persistently mentally ill homeless persons meet the criteria for alcohol or substance dependence. According to the Institute for the Study of Homelessness and Poverty (ISHP 2000), 19–45% of homeless persons are mentally ill and 31–50% have substance use disorders. Among incarcerated females, 72% meet criteria for co-occurring psychiatric illness and substance use disorder (Abram *et al.* 2003). Further, NIDA (2000) reported that 70–90% of all IV drug users are infected with hepatitis C through use of shared needles. This situation is found to lead to significant co-occurring personality and mood alterations (Dieperink *et al.* 2000) as well as depression (Mellors 2000).

Historical context

Prior to the 1980s, diagnosis and treatment of mental illness and substance use disorders in the United States were largely dealt with separately, and little attempt was made to understand and treat them as interactive conditions. It is likely that the paradigm shift in the care of the mentally ill in the early 1980s from deinstitutionalisation to community care contributed to heightening awareness of psychiatric illness co-occurring with substance disorders. As chronically mentally ill persons were transitioned from psychiatric hospitals to community care settings, individuals with primary substance use disorders co-occurring with their mental illnesses and those who used substances as a means to alleviate symptoms of mental illness gained easier access to drugs and alcohol that was previously unavailable in long-term hospitalisation. Clinical evidence of co-occurring psychiatric illness and substance disorders became more apparent and slowly clinicians began to appreciate the interactive nature between the two conditions.

The concept of 'dual diagnosis' was introduced in the United States in the 1980s (Gigliotti 1986; Sciacca 1987a; Thombs 1999). Several terms came into use in the 1980s in the United States to describe dual diagnosis or co-occurring psychiatric illness and substance use disorder. These terms, which were often connected to treatment programmes, include the following:

Dual diagnosis: MICA – mentally ill, chemically addicted; MICAA – mentally ill, chemically addicted and affected; MISA – mentally ill, substance abusing; MISU – mentally ill. Substance using: CAMI – chemically abusing, mentally ill, or chemically addicted, mentally ill; SAMI – substance abusing, mentally ill; MICD – mentally ill, chemically dependent; ICOPSD – individuals with co-occurring psychiatric and substance disorders (Sciacca 1987a, 1987b; Wolf *et al.* 1998; National Library of Medicine, 2001).

During the same time period, the *Diagnostic and Statistical Manual of Mental Disorders III* (American Psychiatric Association 1980), the universally accepted taxonomy for mental health disorders in the United States, introduced the theme of co-occurring disorders by including diagnostic categories for mental illness related to substance use/abuse. This officially recognised the notion of co-occurrence. Research conducted by the National Institute of Mental Health Community Support Program (Ridgely *et al.* 1987) confirmed that individuals with co-occurring psychiatric and substance use disorders could benefit from long-term treatment, thus underscoring the particular needs of this population (Mercer-McFadden *et al.* 1998).

In the 1990s (Sciacca 1991), it was recognised that when clients had co-occurring mental illness and substance use disorders, treatment programmes that were separate and failed to take into account the interaction between the two illnesses proved less effective or ineffective. Gigliotti (1986) and Sciacca (1987a) introduced specific treatment programmes and interventions designed to treat both psychiatric illness and substance disorder co-morbidities simultaneously. These programmes came out of MICA (Mentally ill chemical abusers) models introduced in 1984 to provide simultaneous integrated treatment for those suffering from co-occurring mental illness and substance use disorders and introduced substance disorder interventions into existing programmes for treating major mental illness in order to help clients with both comorbidities.

Currently, the concept of dual diagnosis is widely endorsed in the United States by mental health professionals and substance disorder counsellors. Integrated approaches to treatment that incorporate coordinated, systematic treatment of both co-occurring conditions within one programme are recommended as best practice for dual diagnosis treatment (Shortell *et al.* 2000; Drake *et al.* 2001; SAMHSA 2005; IOM 2005.)

Socio-cultural and public policy considerations

In the United States, all health care has traditionally been funded by health insurance made available through private or public funding sources. Most Americans are covered by health insurance available through their employment (Surgeon General's Report on Mental Health 2000). Currently, such plans include indemnity plans (fee-for-service), and, managed care health plans. Managed care plans purport to offer comprehensive health care services within a framework of cost containment through capitation and primary care 'gatekeeping' wherein primary care clinicians may authorise or deny specialised treatment. Also, Americans over the age of 65 may receive federally funded Medicare health insurance and individual states offer Medicaid health coverage to low-income or indigent individuals and families.

Managed care insurance programmes have created dramatic changes in the organisation and financing of all health care in the United States, with built-in programme incentives towards undertreatment (Murray & Lopez 1996). Quality and accessibility to appropriate mental health care has been affected through cost-containment efforts under managed care. Increased reliance on primary care sources of care service and the introduction of deductibles and co-payments designed to have insured persons share the burden of cost may discourage needed use of mental health services. Under managed healthcare programmes, treatment may be shifted away from in-patient to outpatient care, limiting ideal care options for those who are dually diagnosed (Drake *et al.* 2001). Coverage may extend to programmes that offer dual diagnosis models of treatment, but it is not specifically designated for combined care approaches for individuals who are dually diagnosed.

Although mental health services are covered to some extent by all insurance programmes, there has long existed a lack of parity in coverage for mental health care as compared to care for physical illness, with most insurance companies limiting or restricting mental health coverage (Surgeon General's Report on Mental Health 2000). Currently, legislation is pending at the federal governmental level to mandate parity in insurance coverage funding mental health care, although legislation offered by each House of government differs regarding specific provisions (Trapp 2008), and consensus has been hard to reach. However, eventual parity for mental health care in insurance plans will benefit only those who are eligible and can afford such coverage.

An increasing number of Americans are uncovered by any insurance programme as a result of unemployment, lack of employer-funded insurance coverage or inability to purchase insurance. Seventy-five per cent of these are members of employed families (Surgeon General Report on Mental Health 2000). According to data from the Healthcare for Communities Survey (Watkins *et al.* 2001), 72% of individuals with co-occurring disorders did not receive any substance use or mental health treatment in the past year. Data from 2005 indicate that out of 5.2 million adults with co-occurring mental illness and substance use disorders, 34.3% received treatment only for their mental health disorder, 4.1% received treatment only for their substance use disorder, and 8.5% received treatment for both disorders. Fifty-three per cent received no treatment at all (Center for Substance Abuse Treatment 2007). These statistics may be the result of lack of available services, lack of motivation to access care, inability to access care as a result of lack of insurance coverage or inability to pay or a combination of these factors.

In the United States, there is a pervasive social stigma related to mental illness in general. Moreover, until recently, substance abuse was often considered a moral failing rather than a disease (Center for Addiction and Mental

Health 1999). Hanson (1998) found that the disparity in insurance coverage between mental illness and physical illness serves to further stigmatise this population. Moreover, some clinicians still do not accept the concept of dual diagnosis as co-occurring mental illness and substance use disorders that interact and affect one another. Some maintain the position that psychiatric syndromes are a manifestation of substance use or that substance use is part of a person's psychopathology (Nunes & Rounsaville 2006), which sustains a lack of enthusiasm for dual diagnosis research and treatment initiatives in some clinical circles.

These considerations may account, in part, for the lack of parity and access to care for dual diagnosis in this nation. At present, the health care system in the United States is organizationally and financially complex, uncoordinated and fragmented, creating barriers to research and access to care that can effectively and efficiently manage the complex integrated treatment needs of people with co-occurring mental illness and substance disorders (Drake *et al.* 2001).

Approaches to treatment

It is well recognised that issues related to co-occurring substance use dis orders and major mental illness interact and affect most aspects of treatment for both conditions. Research data demonstrate that individuals with co-occurring mental illness and substance use disorders who receive treatment for both disorders simultaneously have better clinical outcomes (Drake *et al.* 1993; Drake *et al.* 2001; SAMHSA 2005; IOM 2005). Integrated treatment for dual diagnosis is consistent, comprehensive treatment, where both the mental illness and the substance use disorder are treated simultaneously in a coordinated manner with interventions that address both illnesses (Drake *et al.* 2001). In this model of care, health professionals working in one clinical setting provide appropriate treatment for both disorders simultaneously.

The major obstacle to treatment for dually diagnosed individuals is the paucity of available programmes that actually treat both disorders simultaneously in a comprehensive manner. Many care service programmes tend to identify and treat only one of the two co-occurring disorders, leaving the other unrecognised and untreated (Ridgely *et al.* 1990). Addiction professionals and mental health professionals may not view the two co-occurring disorders as separate, yet interrelated, and requiring integrated treatment (Sciacca 1991). This situation creates fragmented, uncoordinated care that can negatively affect care outcomes. If both illnesses are not treated as interrelated, relapse is more probable. Negative outcomes for clients with co-occurring mental illness and substance use disorders include medication non-compliance, relapse, re-hospitalisation, violence, family problems, homelessness, lowered functionality and human immunodeficiency virus (HIV) (Drake & Brunette 1998).

Integrated care models for dual diagnosis treatment work best when they abandon traditional models of substance abuse care that use methods which fail to take into consideration an individual's struggle with co-occurring symptoms of major mental illness. In the United States, these programmes do away with confrontational and moralistic methods in favour of non-judgemental, educational approaches (Sciacca 1991). Sciacca (1991) believes that employing confrontational interventions traditionally used in 12-step programmes for substance use disorders can contribute to possible decompensation in clients with co-occurring major mental illness.

Integrated models welcome individuals even if in denial about one or the other of their co-occurring conditions and they are accepting of all symptoms and experiences relating to both conditions. The treatment focus is on shorter goals because of co-occurring symptoms of major mental illness. The integrated model recognises the ability of symptoms of one condition to affect those of the other; utilises self-help support programmes, and promotes illness education, family involvement and advocacy (Sciacca 1991).

Drake *et al.* (2001) describe best practices in dual diagnosis treatment, based on prior research. Interventions include staged interventions, assertive outreach, motivational interventions, counselling, social support, comprehensiveness and cultural competence and sensitivity in a long-term community-based setting. Assertive outreach, including intensive case management and possible home visits (Mercer-McFadden *et al.* 1998; Ho *et al.* 1999; Drake *et al.* 2001) is especially important for retaining clients within programmes. It is known that without assertive outreach, dropout rates may be high (Hellerstein *et al.* 1995), especially among clients identified as having difficulties participating in treatment, such as homeless persons (Drake *et al.* 2001).

In the United States, there are a variety of treatment programmes available, both in-patient and outpatient, that can operate on a dual diagnosis model. SAMHSA (2006) reported that 35% of substance abuse treatment facilities included programmes or groups for dual diagnosis clients in 2005. These include a variety of care settings to meet specific client needs. These include medically supervised detoxification that usually requires a 3–5 day stay and under the MICA model incorporates assessment of substance condition as well as the mental illness and initiates appropriate treatment for both, including medications, counselling and 12-step model group meetings. Dual diagnosis treatment centres are in-patient programmes that provide integrated, individualised treatment for both illnesses at the same time. These services are individualised and entail a comprehensive programme of stress management, assertive outreach, job and housing assistance, family counselling, money and relationship management and social networking (Cutter *et al.* 2008).

There is a wide array of outpatient treatment services for treatment and management of dual diagnosis symptoms. Some exist within the funded care system in the United States; others are part of the extensive self-help movement in this country. Partial hospitalisation is a programme of 3–5 days in duration, 4–7 hours/day and is usually for individuals who need supervision and monitoring on an outpatient basis. The focus of these programmes is relapse prevention.

Intensive Outpatient Programs (IOP) are relapse prevention programmes scheduled around the individual's work or school timetable and are highly recommended by insurance companies because they are cost effective and have the ability to provide 24-hour coverage (Lehman *et al*. 1997). Clients usually meet 3–5 days a week for 2–4 hours/day. Such initiatives usually fall under the Assertive Community Treatment (ACT) model (Stein & Santos 1998; Coldwell & Bender 2007), first initiated through the efforts of The National Alliance for the Mentally Ill, an important mental health consumer advocacy group in the United States.

There are many peer support or self-help programme options available for people with dual diagnosis. Twelve-step programmes are modelled after the Alcoholics Anonymous model. This self-help group approach has a strong spiritual foundation in which members acknowledge that they are powerless over their addiction and enlist the help of G-d or a 'higher power' to help them manage their lives, based on the individual's own personal belief. Groups are facilitated by fellow addicts where individuals share their stories and knowledge in the context of applying the programme's principles. The meetings are free and the only requirement needed to participate is motivation or a desire to stop abusing substances. However, for those with dual diagnosis, traditional 12-step self-help groups may not meet the complicated needs of those managing both mental illness and substance use disorder simultaneously. To meet this need, Double Trouble in Recovery Groups (www.doubletroubleinrecovery.org) have been founded based on the 12-step model and geared specifically for those dealing with co-occurring symptoms of mental illness and substance use disorders. They address the specific issues people have with managing symptoms of both conditions as interrelated and where each may affect the other. However, there are too few of these groups to meet the needs of all who could benefit from them.

Research

Most research about dual diagnosis in the United States has focused on evaluating clinical treatment programmes that serve clients with co-occurring mental illness and substance use disorders. Early research evaluated the efficacy of adding 12-step substance abuse programmes to traditional treatment programmes for mental illness, and the overall negative outcomes found in this research were considered related to methodological problems in the research and lack of valid and reliable assessment of substance abuse (Drake *et al.* 2001). More recent research has focused on evaluating efficacy of programmes that incorporate assertive outreach, comprehensiveness and long-term rehabilitation approaches and these have produced more optimistic clinical outcomes (Mercer-McFadden *et al.* 1998). Based on their review of the research literature on dual diagnosis, Drake *et al.* (2001) identified several critical components of integrated dual diagnosis programmes that, when present, are associated with positive clinical outcomes and when absent, are predictably associated with poorer outcomes. These include staged treatment interventions, assertive outreach, motivational interventions, counselling, social support interventions, long-term perspective, comprehensiveness and cultural sensitivity and competence (Drake *et al.* 2001). These researchers emphasise the need for outreach and motivational interventions with the dual diagnosis population to enhance attendance and utilisation of treatment programmes.

The research on dual diagnosis in the United States has focused primarily on treatment outcomes within existing programmes; little research has addressed larger issues, such as organization and funding of healthcare services, wider implementation of integrated treatment, training for health care providers and lack of agreement among clinicians about diagnosis and treatment strategies. Also, there is a paucity of research about dual diagnosis in specific vulnerable populations, such as women, homeless persons, impoverished people and individuals with HIV/acquired immmunodeficiency syndrome (AIDS).

Issues and challenges

While the concept of dual diagnosis is supported by research and treatment programmes in the United States, there are still challenges ahead. Most importantly, programmes that treat people with co-occurring mental illness and substance disorders are still far too rare. There is a lack of sufficient programmes to treat everyone needing integrated care and too few professionals with proper educational/training to staff them. This situation is related to several problems in the field. These include multiple barriers in health care policy, financing, regulations and organisational structure currently existing in the United States that result in a lack of collaboration and integration between care delivery systems for mental health disorders and substance disorders (Drake *et al.* 2001). Most treatment for people with co-occurring mental health disorders and substance disorders continues to be handled in separate programmes, usually with one or the other condition ignored or subordinated to care for the other. It is currently recognised that persons with co-occurring disorders may have complex clinical needs that require individualised, respectful, interdisciplinary treatment that stresses collaboration between professionals in 'primary care, human services, housing, criminal justice, education and related fields (SAMHSA/COCE, 2005, p. 3).'

There still appears to be lack of clarity about definitions of dual diagnosis among some mental health clinicians, with issues over proper assessment and diagnosis. Better methods for assessing individuals with co-occurring disorders towards making correct diagnoses that reflect co-occurring conditions are required.

Clinicians need appropriate specialised education to integrate evidence-based best practices into care for dually diagnosed individuals (Annapolis Coalition on the Behavioral Health Workforce 2005). This includes proper assessment and, use of evidence-based, integrated treatment models shown to be associated with optimistic clinical outcome. Appropriate, competent medication management for clients who are managing symptoms of both mental illness and substance disorders is critical to help clients properly manage symptoms of mental illness while simultaneously supporting abstinence from addictive substances. Currently, treatment for co-occurring disorders tends to focus more on mental illness treatment and substance abuse problems are ignored or missed (Drake *et al.* 2001; IOM 2005). Additionally, more research is needed to understand specific needs of dual diagnosis clients with particular vulnerabilities, such as the homeless, the incarcerated, adolescents, individuals with HIV and hepatitis as well as to understand the cultural aspects of co-occurring disorders.

In order to make more integrated treatment programmes for dual diagnosis available, additional governmental funding is needed at both the state and national levels. Public advocacy for funding and initiation of integrated treatment programmes is essential, especially at the community level. Consumers and families need adequate information about co-occurring conditions and the necessity for integrated care programmes to enable them to advocate for programmes to meet the needs of this population. Existing programmes need re-evaluation and upgrading so that they conform to best evidence treatment, moving from more traditional models of care that incorporate interventions that are confrontational and moralistic to treatment models that are non-judgemental, motivational, educational and illness oriented. Self-help organizations based on the 12-step model have always been popular in the United States; however, more groups based on the 'Double-Trouble' philosophy and care model are required to address the kinds of issues people with co-occurring disorders face because traditional 'anonymous' self-help groups are shown to have limited efficacy for this population.

Conclusion

Co-occurring mental illness and substance use disorders are a major public health problem in the United States. The concept of dual diagnosis is well-developed and widely endorsed among researchers and health care providers. Research findings demonstrate the efficacy of integrated long-term programmes for the management of dual diagnosis clients but there is not yet enough public advocacy and governmental attention to support policy, organisational, and funding initiatives to promote more widespread research in the field and availability of integrated programmes for those who need them. Most clients in the United States are still treated for mental illness co-occurring with substance use disorders in separate, unintegrated treatment programmes that ignore or inadequately assess and treat one of the coexisting conditions and/or fail to recognise and consider the interactive nature of the two separate comorbidities and their effect on one another in planning intervention strategies.

References

Abram KA, Teplin LA, McClelland GM (2003) Comorbidity of severe psychiatric disorders and substance abuse among women in jail. *American Journal of Psychiatry* 160 (5): 1007–1010.

American Psychiatric Association (1980) *Diagnostic and Statistical Manual of Mental Disorders-III*. Washington, DC: American Psychiatric Association.

Annapolis Coalition on the Behavioral Health Workforce (2005) Quick Reference Guide To Strategic Goals and Objectives. Retrieved 14.4.2007 from www.annapoliscoalition.org.

Center for Addiction and Mental Health (CAMH) (1999) The Stigma of Substance Use: A Review of the Literature. Retrieved 11.4.2008 from http://www.camh.net/education/Resources_communities_organizations/stigma_subabuse_litreview99.pdf.

Center for Substance Abuse Treatment (2007) *The Epidemiology of Co-occurring Substance Use and Mental Disorders*. COCE Overview, Paper 8, DHHS Publication # SMA 07-4308. Rockville, MD: SAMHSA and Center for Mental Health Services.

Coldwell CM, Bender WS (2007) The effectiveness of assertive community treatment for homeless populations with severe mental illness: A meta-analysis. *American Journal of Psychiatry* 164: 393–399.

Cutter D, Elam S, Jaffe J, Segal J (2008) Dual Diagnosis: Information and Treatment for Co-occurring Disorders. Retrieved 10.4.2008 from www.Helpguide.org/mental/dual_diagnosis.htm.

Dieperink E, Willenbring M, Ho SB (2000) Neuropsychiatric symptoms associated with hepatitis C and interferon alpha: a review. *American Journal of Psychiatry* 157 (6): 867–876.

Drake RE, Bartels SJ, Teague GB, Noordsy DL, Clark RE (1993) Treatment of substance abuse in severely mentally ill patients. *Journal of Nervous and Mental Diseases* 181 (10): 606–611.

Drake RE, Brunette MF (1998) Assessment of substance use among persons with severe mental illness related to alcohol and other drug use disorders. In: Galanter M (ed.). *Consequences of Alcoholism* Vol 14 (pp. 47–78). New York: Plenum.

Drake RE, Essock SM, Shaner A, *et al.* (2001) Implementing dual diagnosis services for clients with severe mental illness. *Psychiatric Services* 52 (4): 469–476.

Gallagher SM, Penn PE, Brooks AJ, Feldman J (2006) Comparing the CAAPE, a new assessment tool for co-occurring disorders, with the SCID. *Psychiatric Rehabilitation Journal* 30 (1): 63–65.

Gigliotti M (1986) *Program Initiatives for Dually-diagnosed at Harlem Valley P.C. Quality of Care Newsletter*, Issue 28, p. 9. New York: New York State Commission on Quality of Care.

Gonzalez G, Rosenheck R (2002) Outcomes and service use among homeless persons with serious mental illness and substance abuse. *Psychiatric Services* 53: 43–46.

Grant B, Stinson F, Dawson D, *et al.* (2004) Prevalence and co-occurrence of substance use disorders and independent mood and anxiety disorders. *Archives of General Psychiatry* 61: 807–816.

Hanson KW (1998) Public opinion and the mental health parity debate: Lessons from the survey literature. *Psychiatric Services* 49: 1059–1066.

Hellerstein DJ, Rosenthal RN, Miner CR (1995) A prospective study of integrated outpatient treatment for substance-abusing schizophrenic patients. *American Journal on Addictions* 4: 33–42.

Ho AP, Tsuang JW, Liberman RP, *et al.* (1999) Achieving effective treatment of patients with chronic psychotic illness and comorbid substance dependence. *American Journal of Psychiatry* 156: 1765–1770.

Institute of Medicine (IOM) (2005) *Improving the Quality of Health Care for Mental and Substance-use Conditions: Quality Chasm Series.* Washington, DC: National Academy Press.

Institute for the Study of Homelessness and Poverty at the Weingart Center (2000) Who is Homeless in Los Angeles? Retrieved 10.3.2008 from http://www.weingart.org/institute/research/facts/pdf/JusttheFacts_LA_Homelessness pdf.

Kessler RC, McGonagle KA, Zhao S, *et al.* (1994) Lifetime and 12 month prevalence of DSM-III-R psychiatric disorders in the United States: Results from the National Comorbidity Survey. *Archives of General Psychiatry* 51: 8–9.

Lehman AF, Dixon LB, Kernan E, DeForge BR, Postrado LT (1997) A randomized trial of assertive community treatment for homeless persons with severe mental illness. *Archives of General Psychiatry* 54: 1038–1043.

Mellors D (2000) Hepatitis C and Depression. Hepatitis C Review, 30. Retrieved 13.3.2008 from http://www.hepatitisc.org.au/reviews/current_editions/edition30.htm.

Mercer-McFadden C, Drake RE, Clark RE, Verven N, Noordsy DL, Fox TS (1998) *Substance Abuse Treatment for People with Severe Mental Disorders: A Program Manager's Guide.* Concord, NH: New Hampshire-Dartmouth Psychiatric Research Center.

Murray C, Lopez A (1996) *The Global Burden of Disease.* Cambridge, MA: Harvard University Press.

National Institute on Drug Abuse (2000) Community Drug Alert Bulletin: Hepatitis C. (NIDA Booklet. NCADI#PHD838). Retrieved 10.3.2008 from http://165.112.78.61/HepatitisAlert/HepatitisAlert.html.

National Library of Medicine (NLM) (2001) Health Services/Technology Assessment Text. AHCPR Archived reports. Put prevention into practice and Minnesota Health Committee. SAMHSA/CSAT Treatment Improvement Protocols, 42 TIP 42. Substance Abuse Treatment for Persons with Co-occurring Disorders. Retrieved 13.2.2008 from http://www.ncbi.nlm.nih.gov/books/bv.fcgi?rid=hstat5.section.74165.

Nunes EV, Rounsaville BJ (2006) Comorbidity of substance use with depression and other mental disorders: from diagnostic and statistical manual of mental disorders (DSM-IV) to DSM-V. *Addiction* 101 (Suppl. 1): 89–96.

President's New Freedom Commission on Mental Health (2003) Achieving the Promise: Transforming Mental Health Care in America. Retrieved 9.4.2008 from http://www.mentalhealthcommission.gov/index.html.

Ridgely MS, Goldman HH, Willenbring M (1990) Barriers to the care of persons with dual diagnosis: Organizational and financing issues. *Schizophrenia Bulletin* 16: 123–132.

Ridgely MS, Osher FC, Goldman HH (1987) *Chronic Mentally Ill Young Adults with Substance Abuse Problems: A Review of Research, Treatment and Training Issues. Report of the Department of Psychiatry Task Force on Chronic Mentally Ill Young adults with Substance Problems.* Baltimore, MD: University of Maryland.

SAMHSA (Substance Abuse and Mental Health Services Administration) (2004) *Results from the 2003 National Survey on Drug Use and Health: National Findings.* Rockville, MD: SAMHSA DHHS Publication No (SMA) 04-3966.

SAMHSA (Substance Abuse and Health Services Administration) (2005) Transforming Mental Health Care in America: The Federal Action Agenda: First Steps. Retrieved 10.4.2008 from www.samhsa.gov/federalactionagenda/NFCTOC.aspx.

SAMHSA/COCE (2005) Overarching principles to address the needs of persons with co-occurring disorders. COCE overview paper 3. DHHS Pub. (SMA) 06-4165. Rockville, MD: Substance Abuse and Mental Health Services Administration.

SAMHSA/DASIS. Substance Abuse and Mental Health Services Administration/Drug and Alcohol Services Information System (2006) The

DASIS Report: Facilities Offering Special Programs or Groups for Clients with Co-occurring Disorders: 2004. Retrieved 10.4.2008 from www.oas. samhsa.gov.

Sciacca K (1987a) Alcohol and substance abuse programs at New York state psychiatric centers. *Develop and Expand ... AID Bulletin Addiction Intervention with the Disabled* 9 (2): 1–3.

Sciacca K (1987b) New Initiatives in the Treatment of the Chronic Patient with Alcohol/Substance Use Problems. TIE Lines, 4(3). Information Exchange of Young Adult Chronic Patients.

Sciacca K (1991) *An Integrated Treatment Approach for Severely Mentally Ill Individuals with Substance Disorders. New Directions for Mental Health Services*, Ch 6. San Francisco, CA: Jossey-Bass.

Shortell SM, Gillies RR, Anderson DA, Erickson KM, Mitchell JB (2000) *Remaking Health Care in America: The Evolution of Organized Delivery Systems*, 2nd Edition. San Francisco, CA: Jossey-Bass.

Stein LI, Santos AB (1998) *Assertive Community Treatment of Persons with Severe Mental Illness*. New York: Norton.

Surgeon General's Report on Mental Health (2000) Washington, DC: US Government Printing Office.

Thombs DL (1999) *Introduction to Addictive Behaviors*, 2nd Edition. New York: Guilford Press.

Trapp D (2008) Parity, genetic privacy bills face snag. *American Medical News* 51 (8): American Medical Association. Retrieved from http://www.ama. assn.org/amednews/2008/02/25/gvsa0225.htm.

Watkins KE, Burnam A, Kung FY, Paddock S (2001) A national survey of care for persons with co-occurring mental and substance use disorders. *Psychiatry Services* 52 (8): 1062–1068.

Wolf AW, Schubert DS, Patterson MB, Grande TP, Brocco KJ, Pendleton L (1998) Association among psychiatric diagnosis. *Journal of Consulting and Clinical Psychology* 56: 292–294.

Chapter 19

Dual Diagnosis – Australasia

Gary Croton

Introduction

This chapter outlines some of the drivers for system change in regard to Australian treatment systems' recognition of and response to co-occurring mental health and substance use disorders (dual diagnosis). It describes some of the Australian barriers to achieving better outcomes for persons with dual diagnosis as well as the special needs of Indigenous Australians and people living in rural and remote regions of Australia. The chapter concludes with a summary of some of the main, current Australian initiatives addressing the various treatment systems' recognition of and response to the needs of persons presenting with dual diagnosis. While the term 'dual diagnosis' is used to refer to co-occurring mental health and substance use disorders, the terms 'comorbidity', 'coexisting disorders', 'concurrent disorders' and 'co-occurring disorders' may be substituted at the reader's preference.

Drivers for system change

In Australia, as in the rest of the Western world, co-occurring mental health and substance use disorders are highly prevalent, especially so in persons receiving treatment for either a mental health or a substance use disorder. Table 1 summarises some of the available data on the prevalence of co-occurring mental health and substance use disorder in Australia.

Consumer and carer demand

Mental health consumers and carer peak bodies have identified developing more effective responses to the needs of persons with both disorders as one of the top two priorities for mental health services in Australia (MHCA 2005).

The 2006/07 Australian Senate Mental Health Inquiry, which took extensive submissions from a host of mental health consumers, carers and their representative organisations, devoted the greatest part of its comprehensive report to dual diagnosis (Senate Select Committee on Mental Health 2006).

Prevalence

Co-occurring mental health and substance use disorders are highly prevalent in Australia, especially in persons receiving treatment for either a mental health or a substance use disorder. Table 19.1 summarises some of the available data on the prevalence of co-occurring mental health and substance use disorder in Australia.

Harms and unwanted outcomes strongly associated with dual diagnosis

There is a substantial body of literature that documents the harms and unwanted outcomes strongly associated with dual diagnosis. These include more frequent relapse and hospitalisation (Cuffel & Chase 1994), increased treatment costs (Hoff & Rosenheck 1999), greater housing difficulties and homelessness (Lipton *et al.* 2000), exposure to violence and exploitation (Sells *et al.* 2003), forensic involvement (Wallace *et al.* 2004) and physical disorders (Dickey *et al.* 2002).

While most of the research interest to date has focused on the harms associated with severe mental health disorders co-occurring with severe substance use disorders, it is worth noting that the bulk of harms and costs associated with substance use disorders is attributable to the large cohort of persons who meet the criteria for substance abuse rather than the smaller, more visible cohort that meets the criteria for substance dependence. If the same holds true for costs and harms associated with the large cohort of persons who meet the criteria for high-prevalence, lower impact mental health disorders (where, as with substance abuse, treatment is lower input and more effective) then it is likely that the greatest financial and social savings may be realised by increasing the investment in service systems, increasing their recognition of and providing treatment to the large cohort of persons with less severe substance use disorders co-occurring with less severe substance use disorders. Note that Hickie *et al.*, in 2001, found co-occurring mental disorders and substance misuse in 12% of patients attending general practice for any reason ($n = 46,515$).

Table 19.1   Australian estimates of prevalence of dual diagnosis

Prevalence in the general population	The last 15–20 years has seen a number of nations fund large-scale studies to ascertain the prevalence of mental health disorders in the general population. The Australian version, the 1997 National Survey of Mental Health and Wellbeing (NSMHW), was a household survey that assessed a representative sample of 10,641 respondents for symptoms of high-prevalence mental health disorders including substance use disorders.

The NSMHW found that, in any 12-month period

- 9.7% of the population met criteria for an anxiety disorder
- 7.7% met the criteria for a substance use disorder and
- 5.8% met the criteria for an affective (mood) disorder

(Andrews *et al*. 1999)

In regard to dual diagnosis, the NSMHW data revealed that one in four of the persons with one of the above common (high-prevalence) disorders also had one of the other disorders.

- In females, while only 15% of females without an alcohol use disorder had any mental disorder, 48% of those with an alcohol use disorder also met criteria for an anxiety, affective or drug use disorder.
- In males, while only 9% of males without an alcohol use disorder had a mental disorder, 34% of those with an alcohol use disorder had another mental disorder (Teeson *et al*. 2000).
- Alcohol-dependent persons were 4.5 times more likely than other Australians to also have an affective disorder.
- Alcohol-dependent persons were 4.4 times more likely than other Australians to also have an anxiety disorder.
- Cannabis-dependent persons were 4.3 times more likely than other Australians to also have an anxiety disorder.
- Tobacco users were 2.2 times more likely to also have an affective disorder.
- Tobacco users were 2.4 times more likely to also have an anxiety disorder (Degenhardt *et al*. 2001).
- 180,000 men and 130,000 women (310,000 Australians) had a substance use disorder co-occurring with either an anxiety or a affective disorder in the previous 12 months (Kavanagh 2003).
- Of persons with an alcohol use disorder in the previous 12 months, 18% also had an affective disorder and 15% also had an anxiety disorder.
- Of persons with an affective disorder in the previous 12 months, 17% also had an alcohol use disorder.
- Of persons with an anxiety disorder in the previous 12 months, 16% also had an alcohol use disorder (Burns *et al*. 2001).

Table 19.1 *(continued)*

Prevalence in persons in primary care	The high prevalence of co-occurring disorders in the general population data reported above has relevance to the prevalence of co-occurring disorders in primary care settings – in 2000–2001, the average Australian had between four and six consultations with a general practitioner (GP) or specialist (AIHW 2004). A 2001 study by Hickie *et al.* examined the comorbidity of common mental disorders and alcohol or other substance misuse in Australian general practice (*n* = 46,515) and found overall prevalence of mental health and/or substance use among persons attending general practice of 56%. Co-occurring mental disorders and substance misuse in 12% of patients attending general practice. (Hickie *et al.* 2001)
Prevalence in persons receiving treatment for a mental health disorder	The 1997 NSMHW also conducted a low-prevalence survey examining aspects of the lives of persons with psychosis (*n* = 970). (Jablensky *et al.* 1999). This survey painted a grim picture of the quality of life of persons with psychosis in Australia and evidence of very high rates of co-occurring substance use disorders. • 40% of persons with psychosis met lifetime criteria for substance abuse or dependence • 17.4% met criteria for abuse or dependence on two or more substances • 70% of the sample had or had had a substance use disorder involving nicotine • 27% involving alcohol • 22% involving cannabis and • 12% 'other substances' (Kavanagh *et al.* 2004) Victorian Mental Health Branch 2002 telephone survey (*n* = 1858): In 2002, the Victorian Mental Health Branch conducted a telephone survey of persons receiving treatment from Victorian mental health services. Despite methodology likely to lead to underreporting, the survey found that 45% of persons receiving acute mental health treatment reported a co-occurring alcohol or drug abuse/dependence problem.
Prevalence in persons receiving treatment for a substance use disorder	In a 2001 study of the prevalence of psychiatric disorders in persons recently entering a methadone maintenance programme (*n* = 62), *Callaly et al.* (2001) found that in the 12 months prior to interview: • more than 50% met criteria for an affective disorder • two-thirds fulfilled criteria for an anxiety disorder • just under half met criteria for both an affective disorder and an anxiety disorder

(continued)

Table 19.1 *(continued)*

	At the time of interview:
	• 19% met criteria for a moderate or severe affective disorder
	• 70% of males and 89% of females had a co-morbid psychiatric illness
	• 71% of the group with comorbidity reported that onset of psychiatric symptomatology predated the use of heroin
	• The prevalence of psychiatric disorder is up to 10 times higher in the population on methadone maintenance than in the general population and is 2–3 times higher than that found in community surveys of those with a substance-use disorder
Forensic populations	Australian researchers Wallace *et al.* (2004) found striking evidence of the contribution made by co-occurring substance abuse to the likelihood that persons with schizophrenia will commit criminal offences. They compared the criminal records of patients with a first admission for schizophrenia in Victoria in 1975, 1980, 1985, 1990 and 1995 ($n = 2861$) with those of an equal number of community comparison subjects matched for age, gender and neighbourhood of residence. They found that persons with schizophrenia committed nearly eight times the number of offences as the non-schizophrenia matched control group and also that much higher rates of criminal conviction were found for persons with schizophrenia with substance abuse problems than for those without substance abuse problems (68.1% versus 11.7%).
	Ogloff *et al.* (2004) study of the prevalence in forensic mental health treatment settings found that 74% of patients had a lifetime substance abuse or dependence disorder (and also that the patients with substance use disorders had more extensive criminal histories, had more complex needs and posed more risks than clients with mental illness alone).

Opportunity to provide more effective treatment of 'target' disorders via improved recognition and more effective responses to co-occurring disorders

Co-occurring mental health and substance use disorders will, in any individual experiencing them, influence each other in their development, their severity, their response to treatment and their relapse circumstances. Hence any treatment provided for one of the disorders in isolation, treatment that fails to recognise or respond to any co-occurring disorder, is much less likely to be successful. The corollary of this is that treatment that does recognise the presence of a co-occurring disorder and provides or facilitates evidence-based treatment for all presenting disorders is more likely to be successful.

Contextual issues

This section will describe some of the Australian barriers to achieving better outcomes for persons with dual diagnosis and briefly review the particular challenges faced by Indigenous Australians and people living in rural and remote regions of Australia.

Barriers to better outcomes for persons with dual diagnosis

Australia, along with much of the Western world, experiences significant systemic and other barriers to more effectively addressing co-occurring disorders. Australian researchers (Kavanagh *et al.* 2000) surveyed staff from both mental health and drug treatment services in order to determine their opinions and experiences in treating persons with co-occurring disorders. Issues raised as substantial problems included lack of specialised services, poor coordination of mental health and drug treatment services and frustrations with attempting to provide clinical services to this client group. In other Australian research, Szirom *et al.* (2004) examined barriers to service provision for young people presenting with substance misuse and mental health problems. Identified barriers included the following:

- Homelessness
- Challenging, volatile or violent behaviour
- Appointment-based service provision
- Definitional difficulties
- Lack of specialist services and dedicated resources
- Lack of expertise and dual skills
- Conflicting interests in service provision

Croton (2005) identified the following factors that may contribute to mental health and/or drug treatment worker's ambivalence around addressing co-occurring disorders:

- Perception of added work rather than more effective work
- Lack of awareness of prevalence, harms, relationships between disorders and treatment implications
- 'Therapeutic nihilism' – lack of confidence in the effectiveness of 'the opposite' treatment approaches

- Lack of skills and knowledge in deploying drug treatment or mental health treatment approaches
- Implication of current 'wrong practice'
- Changes to practice, language, beliefs, values, exclusion criteria
- May be a change-weary and change-wary group
- Stigma of client group – two relapsing highly stigmatised disorders in one individual
- Clinicians' own cognitive dissonance (to address my client's substance use or mental health issue it is necessary, at some level, to examine my own substance use or mental health issues)
- History of own substance-related or mental health-related trauma
- Lack of knowledge of the 'opposite' treatment system and the constraints on the extent of service possible from that system

Indigenous Australians

Indigenous, Aboriginal and Torres Strait Islander people represent 2.5% of the total Australian population. On nearly all health and social indicators, Indigenous Australians experience significantly worse outcomes than non-Indigenous Australians. Indigenous life expectancy is on average 17 years less and mortality rates are three times that of non-Indigenous Australians. Indigenous Australians suffer a burden of disease that is two-and-a-half times greater than the burden of disease in the total Australian population. Indigenous Australians experience three times greater unemployment rates, have median household incomes less than 60% of non-Indigenous Australians, have half the home ownership rates and one quarter live in overcrowded housing situations (Pink & Allbon 2008). For many Indigenous Australians, multiple, co-occurring problems and disorders are the rule rather than the exception.

In regard to Indigenous substance use, while in 2004–2005 Indigenous Australians were more likely than non-Indigenous Australians to be alcohol abstinent,

- Indigenous Australians have higher rates of binge drinking than non-Indigenous Australians in every age group (Pink & Allbon 2008);
- Indigenous Australians were twice as likely to drink at short-term risky/high-risk levels at least once a week (Pink & Allbon 2008);
- in 2003, alcohol was associated with 7% of all deaths and 6% of the total burden of disease for Indigenous Australians (Vos *et al.* 2007);
- excessive alcohol consumption accounted for the greatest proportion of the burden of disease and injury for young Indigenous males (Pink & Allbon 2008);

- there is twice the rate of regular smokers among the Indigenous population (Pink & Allbon 2008).
  In regard to Indigenous mental health and social and emotional well-being,
- Indigenous adults are twice as likely to report high levels of psychological distress;
- Indigenous adults were twice as likely as non-Indigenous adults to have reported mental illness as a stressor;
- in 2005–2006, hospitalisations for 'mental and behavioural disorders due to psychoactive substance use' were almost five times higher for Indigenous males and around three times higher for Indigenous females;
- in 2005–2006, Indigenous Australian males were three times more likely to be hospitalised for intentional self-harm than non-Indigenous Australians; Indigenous females were twice as likely (Pink & Allbon 2008).

Rural and remote regions of Australia

Thirty percent of the Australian population lives in either rural or remote regions. In general, Australian health outcomes worsen with increasing rurality. Persons living in metropolitan settings have greater longevity and higher health standards than their rural counterparts. Even when lower socio-economic status is factored in rural health, outcomes are worse than metropolitan.

While there are large research gaps in regard to metropolitan/rural dual diagnosis differences there is evidence for the following:

- The prevalence of common mental health disorders is largely similar between metropolitan and rural regions (Eckert *et al*. 2004).
- Alcohol use disorders, for some age cohorts, are more prevalent in rural areas – rural males and females in the 20–29 years age group are twice as likely to consume alcohol in hazardous or harmful quantities.
- Suicide rates increase with increasing rurality (Caldwell *et al*. 2004). Suicide rates are increasing, especially for males in inland towns with populations of less than 4000. Completed suicide for men in the 15–24 years cohort in remote areas is 43 per 100,000 against 24 per 100,000 in capital cities (Moon *et al*. 1999).
- With increasing remoteness young males are less likely to report a mental health disorder and less likely to seek help for a mental health disorder (Caldwell *et al*. 2004).

Table 19.2 summarises some of the factors commonly identified as underpinning rural Australia's worse health outcomes.

Table 19.2 Factors commonly identified as underpinning rural Australia's worse health outcomes

Service access	Lack of the full range of services ● especially specialised services ● especially in crisis response ● Travel time and costs ● financial and opportunity costs for persons needing to travel to access services ● financial and time costs for services to outreach to persons in remote areas
Structural	Aboriginal and Torres Strait Islander, aged and adolescents cohorts – are all proportionally higher in rural and remote regions **Environmental hazards –** the impacts of drought, flood, fire and changed farming conditions are much greater in rural and remote regions
Attitudinal	Stigma Confidentiality may be harder to maintain in a smaller community where 'dual relationships' (professional and personal) are more common Stoicism – rural persons less likely to report or seek help for problems Risk taking
Workforce	**Shortages and misdistribution favouring urban areas –** for instance, while 30% of the population lives in rural or remote regions, only 4% of psychiatrists and 12% of psychologists practice in those regions Rural workforce shortages lead to ● patients lacking choice in mental health care providers ● providers tending to focus more on more severe mental health and substance use disorders (where treatment tends to be higher-input and less effective) rather than less severe mental health and substance use disorders (where treatment tends to be lower-input and more effective) ● GPs being overburdened because of a lack of other mental health professionals Rural worker tensions include ● maintaining confidentiality and managing 'dual' relationships ● access to education and training and clinical supervision ● professional isolation ● stigma of rural practice ● multiple demands on workers that may be outside their training and expertise

Australia's responses to dual diagnosis

This section briefly describes the structure of the Australian health care system before outlining some of the main, current Australian initiatives addressing the various treatment systems' recognition of and response to the needs of persons presenting with dual diagnosis. This summary was compiled in 2008 – readers should be aware that this is a rapidly changing environment with frequent new initiatives and developments at the systemic, agency, clinician and research community levels.

Structure of the Australian health care system

Australia has eight states and territories – the Australian Capital Territory, New South Wales, the Northern Territory, Queensland, South Australia, Tasmania, Victoria and Western Australia. Each state government has primary responsibility for the state's health system regulating and funding the general hospitals and community health services. The federal (Commonwealth) government has an overarching role in providing funding to the states, defining policy and setting health care objectives and in funding a universal health safety net through the 'Medicare' system.

National level responses to dual diagnosis

The Commonwealth's preferred term for co-occurring mental health and substance use disorders is *comorbidity*. At the national Australian level, the most significant responses to dual diagnosis to date have been as follows:

- The National Comorbidity Initiative (NCI)
- Improved Services for People with Drug and Alcohol Problems and Mental Illness measure
- 'Can Do' – Managing Mental Health and Substance Use in General Practice
- Headspace

The National Comorbidity Initiative

The Australian Government allocated $17.9 million for 2003–2010 to improve service coordination and treatment outcomes for persons with comorbidity. The NCI has directed the bulk of it's investment in developing the response to comorbidity in the alcohol and other drug (AOD) and general practice sectors.

The NCI prioritises the following:

- Raising health workers' awareness of comorbidity and promoting examples of good practice
- Supporting GPs and other health workers to improve treatment outcomes
- Improving consumer's access to resources and information
- Improving data systems within mental health and AOD sectors to manage dual diagnosis more effectively

Completed projects include the following:

- Analysis of general practice encounter databases: key finding that persons with substance use disorders were at twice the risk of developing depressive disorders compared to the non-substance users
- Qualitative treatment experience study: research to identify barriers and incentives to treatment experienced by persons with dual diagnosis, identify treatment options and develop policy and programme level recommendations. See the report at http://www.nationaldrugstrategy. gov.au/internet/drugstrategy/publishing.nsf/Content/mono61
- Consumer and carer involvement in comorbidity treatment planning: study examining the benefits of involving consumers and carers in comorbidity treatment planning processes that led to the development of a 'Consumer and Carer Involvement in Comorbidity Treatment Planning Package'
- Review of current data collections databases: a report on the current state of data collections relevant to people with comorbidity. See http://www.aihw.gov.au/publications/index.cfm/title/10132

Current projects include the following:

- Service model evaluation: an evaluation of 15 service delivery models for comorbidity treatment in the AOD and mental health sectors with the aim of identifying good practice models. The evaluation is expected to be completed in May 2009.
- Comorbidity Professional Development Scholarships Program: offers non-government AOD and mental health organisations and their staff professional development scholarships to build their expertise in the detection and treatment of mental health and substance use disorders – see http://www.nceta.flinders.edu.au/projects/comorbidity.html
- 'Can Do' – Managing Mental Health and Substance Use in General Practice: described below.
- PsyCheck: Developed out of a Commonwealth Department of Health and Aging multi-site implementation process, PsyCheck is a mental

health screening tool and treatment package designed to assist AOD workers to identify and respond to co-occurring mental health disorders. PsyCheck is currently being disseminated nationally – see http://www.psycheck.org.au/

- National Comorbidity Clinical Guidelines: targeting the AOD sector, these guidelines will describe good practice in responding to co-occurring mental health disorders.
- Clinical Supervision of Psychologists and Social Workers in AOD training placements: this initiative will fund clinical supervision of psychologists and social workers in AOD training placements with the aim of exposing them to AOD work early in their careers as well as building their dual diagnosis recognition and treatment expertise.
- Review of comorbidity of mental disorders and substance use: Brief Guide for the primary care clinician: due to be completed in June 2008.
- Clinical review of Dual Diagnosis Primary Care Guide: due to be completed in July 2008.

Improved Services for People with Drug and Alcohol Problems and Mental Illness Measure

The Australian Government Department of Health and Ageing allocated $65.7 million, for the 5 years from July 2007, to the Improved Services measure. The Improved Services measure aims to build the capacity of non-government drug and alcohol treatment services to better identify and treat clients with coinciding drug and alcohol problems and mental illness. Capacity building grants have been allocated, via a competitive grant process, to non-government drug and alcohol treatment services across Australia to undertake a range of capacity building activities including workforce training, developing partnerships with local area health services and developing and implementing policies and procedures that support the identification and management of clients experiencing comorbidity.

A component of the Improved Services funding was directed to Cross Sectorial Support and Strategic Partnerships Projects (CSSSP) in each state. These projects funded each state's AOD peak body to support the capacity building grant recipients and to coordinate a statewide approach to the projects.

'Can Do' – Managing Mental Health and Substance Use in General Practice

Launched in late 2006, under the auspices of the Australian General Practice Network and funded as part of the NCI, 'Can Do' aims to build awareness, clinical knowledge and skills in management and treatment of dual diagnosis in the general practice setting. 'Can Do' focuses on education, training and networking between two multidisciplinary teams of health professionals: general practice teams and community health teams (especially those engaged in alcohol and drug service, community pharmacy and mental health service delivery).

'Can Do' now comprises several components including Teams of Two, Clinical Education and eight population-specific modules. See http://www.agpncando.com/.

Headspace

Launched in 2006, auspiced by a coalition of the Australian Division of General Practice, ORYGEN Research Centre, the Australian Psychological Society and the Brain and Mind Research Institute, Headspace is a $54 million initiative that aims to reduce the burden of disease in young people aged 12–25 years caused by mental health and related substance use.

Headspace's chief strategy is to fund the development of 'Communities of Youth Services' (CYS). CYSs are partnerships of health, education and welfare service providers working to reform their response to young people with mental health and related substance use issues.

Key CYS activities include the following:

- The delivery of community awareness campaigns to their local community that build the likelihood that young persons will seek help as well as local service providers' and families' capacity to identify emerging mental health concerns
- Developing specialist, youth and carer-friendly CYSs to ensure that young people's needs are met with a coordinated and integrated response.
- Use of Headspace training packages to strengthen local mental health, primary care and other workers' use of evidence-based approaches in mental health care
- Linking young people into appropriate vocational and educational supports
- Engaging young people and carers in the development of their local headspace service platform

Headspace has established a centre of excellence research facility charged with identifying and disseminating evidence-based practice in addressing youth mental health issues. Headspace's focus is on evidenced-based approaches, early intervention, access to treatment, overcoming stigma around youth mental illness, improving the professional training of mental health workers and understanding the links between mental health and drug and alcohol abuse. More information can be found at http://www.headspace.org.au/.

State level responses to dual diagnosis

All Australian states have implemented some initiatives addressing dual diagnosis. Since 1998, Victoria has devoted the most significant resources and attention to achieving better outcomes for persons with dual diagnosis.

Victoria's responses to dual diagnosis

In 1998, the Victorian Department of Human Services (DHS) established the Substance Use Mental Illness Treatment Team (SUMITT) pilot in the western regions of Melbourne and rural Victoria. This pilot project was charged with providing direct clinical services and capacity building with both AOD and mental health services. Learnings from this project informed the 2002 establishment of the cross-sector planned and funded statewide initiative Victorian Dual Diagnosis Initiative (VDDI). VDDI workers, in each region of the state, were also given responsibility for capacity building and providing direct clinical services. VDDI capacity was augmented in 2002 by the creation of dedicated youth dual diagnosis specialist positions. The years 2005 and 2006 saw the creation of the following:

- The Rotations project: Under this project interested AOD or mental health workers were funded to undertake a 3-month rotation in the 'other' sector as the hub of a 12-month staff development and education process. This ongoing project has been evaluated and has built the capacity of both AOD and mental health sectors to respond effectively to persons with dual diagnosis.
- The VDDI Statewide Dual Diagnosis Education and Training Unit (the VDDI E&T Unit): The unit has developed nationally recognised diploma level dual diagnosis competencies that are being delivered by a number of education providers through online and face-to-face delivery. The VDDI E&T Unit has also developed dual diagnosis subjects for postgraduate courses through universities and private higher education providers.

The year 2006 also saw

- at state government level, the establishment of a dedicated Minister for Mental Health and Drugs;
- at the central policy and planning level, the merger of the former Mental Health Branch and the Drugs Policy Branch into the Division of Mental Health and Drugs.

In 2007, the Minister for Mental Health and Drugs launched the cross-sector policy 'Dual diagnosis: key directions and priorities for service development policy' (Victorian Government 2007). This policy described the next steps to be taken in improving the provision of treatment and care to persons presenting with dual diagnosis to both specialist mental health and AOD services. The policy contained five service development outcomes, each with key performance indicators and timelines, for mental health and AOD services to work towards.

Particular strengths of the Victorian policy include that it

- was designed around both mental health and AOD treatment sectors;
- mandated that responding to dual diagnosis was 'core business' for both mental health and AOD services and clinicians;
- built in consumer and carer input;
- focused on achieving agency and clinician 'dual diagnosis capability';
- prioritised and articulated a workable definition of integrated treatment;
- prioritised the development of a 'no wrong door' service system;
- allocated broad treatment responsibility for the various cohorts of persons with dual diagnosis (primary care/specialist AOD/specialist mental health).

Reporting on the service's progress to date in achieving the service development outcomes indicates rapid development in specialist service's capacity to respond effectively to persons with dual diagnosis.

Other states' responses to dual diagnosis

The various Australian states and territories all experience unique opportunities and challenges in developing more effective responses to the treatment needs of persons with dual diagnosis. Queensland has, since 2004, had a number of specialist dual diagnosis workers across the state building workers' and service's capacity and is soon to roll out a statewide dual diagnosis policy that will be supported by dual diagnosis 'champions' embedded in specialist treatment services. South Australia and Tasmania also have had specialist dual diagnosis workers for some time.

New South Wales has long had an elegant AOD assessment form embedded into their statewide routine mental health assessment documentation suite and recently released a Mental Health Resource Guideline for Drug and Alcohol Workers (http://www.health.nsw.gov.au/pubs/2007/mh_resource.html), a resource kit for GPs managing comorbidity in the community (http://www.health.nsw.gov.au/resources/drugsandalcohol/

patientjourneykit2_pdf.asp) and a NSW Health Mental Health/Drug and Alcohol Comorbidity Framework for Action (http://www.health.nsw.gov.au/pubs/2008/comorbidity_frame.html).

Conclusion

While the Australian health care system already has substantial achievements around evolving systemic dual diagnosis capability, there is also widespread recognition of the long journey ahead before we can be confident that our service systems are offering the most effective possible responses to persons presenting with dual diagnosis.

There is a need for greater alignment of national mental health and alcohol and drug planning processes, recognition of the likely large-scale gains and savings achievable by an increased focus on the large cohort of persons with high-prevalence mental health disorders co-occurring with substance abuse rather than dependence and a recognition that, because of the much greater numbers of persons who receive treatment in mental health systems, that a focus on developing the most effective possible responses in mental health systems should also be a national priority.

References

Andrews G, Hall W, Teesson M, Henderson S (1999) *National Survey of Mental Health and Wellbeing: Report 2: The Mental Health of Australians.* Canberra: Department of Health and Aged Care.

Australian Institute of Health and Welfare (AIHW) (2004) *Australia's Health 2004.* Canberra: AIHW.

Burns C, Lynskey M, Teesson M (2001) The Epidemiology of Comorbidity between Alcohol Use Disorders and Mental Disorders in Australia. Technical Report No. 118. Sydney: National Drug and Alcohol Research Centre, University of New South Wales.

Caldwell T, Jorm A, Dear K (2004) Suicide and mental health in rural, remote and metropolitan areas in Australia. *Medical Journal of Australia* 181 (7): 10–14. http://www.mja.com.au/public/issues/181_07_041004/suppl_contents_041004.html, http://www.mja.com.au/public/issues/181_07_041004/cal10801_fm.pdf.

Callaly T, Trauer T, Munro L, Whelan G (2001) Prevalence of psychiatric disorder in a methadone maintenance population. *Australian and New Zealand Journal of Psychiatry* 35: 601–605.

Croton G (2005) *Senate Mental Health Inquiry Submission: Australian Treatment System's Recognition of and Response to Co-occurring Mental Health & Substance Use Disorders.* Eastern Hume Dual Diagnosis Service.

Cuffel BJ, Chase P (1994) Remission and relapse of substance use disorders in schizophrenia: Results from a one year prospective study. *Journal of Nervous and Mental Disease* 182: 342–348.

Degenhardt L, Hall W, Lynskey M (2001) Alcohol, cannabis and tobacco use among Australians: a comparison of their associations with other drug use and use disorders, affective and anxiety disorders and psychosis. *Addiction* 96: 1603–1614.

Dickey B, Normand S-LT, Weiss RD, Drake RE, Azeni H (2002) Medical morbidity, mental illness, and substance use disorders. *Psychiatric Services* 53: 861–867.

Eckert K, Taylor A, Wilkinson D, Tucker G (2004) How does mental health status relate to accessibility and remoteness? *Medical Journal of Australia* 181 (10): 540–543.

Hickie I, Koschera A, Davenport T, Naismith S, Scott E (2001) Comorbidity of common mental disorders and alcohol or other substance misuse in Australian general practice. *Medical Journal of Australia* 175: S31–S36.

Hoff RA, Rosenheck RA (1999) The cost of treating substance abuse patients with and without comorbid psychiatric disorders. *Psychiatric Services* 50 (10): 1309–1315.

Jablensky A, McGrath J, Herrman H, *et al.* (1999) *National Survey of Mental Health and Wellbeing, Report 4. People Living with Psychotic Illness: An Australian Study 1997–8 an overview*. Canberra: Department of Health and Aged Care.

Kavanagh DJ (2003) Social and Economic Costs of Comorbid Substance Abuse and Mental Disorder. Submission to the 2003 House of Representatives Standing Committee on Family and Community Affairs Inquiry into Substance Abuse in Australian Communities.

Kavanagh DJ, Greenaway L, Jenner L, *et al.* (2000) Contrasting views and experiences of health professionals on the management of comorbid substance use and mental health disorders. *Australian and New Zealand Journal of Psychiatry* 34: 279–289.

Kavanagh DJ, Waghorn G, Jenner L, *et al.* (2004) Demographic and clinical correlates of comorbid substance use disorders in psychosis: multivariate analyses from an epidemiological sample. *Schizophrenia Research* 66: 115–124.

Lipton FR, Siegel C, Hannigan A, Samuels J, Baker S (2000) Tenure in supportive housing for homeless persons with severe mental illness. *Psychiatric Services* 51: 479–486.

Mental Health Council of Australia (MHCA) website. Fact Sheet Top 25 Community Priorities http://www.mhca.com.au/Public/FactSheets/Top25CommunityPriorities1to10.html (Accessed May 2005).

Moon L, Meyer P, Grau J (1999) *Australia's Young People: Their Health and Well-being*. PHE 19. Canberra: Australian Institute of Health and Welfare.

Ogloff J, Lemphers A, Dwyer C (2004) Dual diagnosis in an Australian forensic psychiatric hospital: prevalence and implications for services. *Behavioural Sciences and the Law* 22 (4): 543–562.

Pink B, Allbon P (2008) *The Health and Welfare of Australia's Aboriginal and Torres Strait Islander Peoples 2008*. Canberra: Australian Bureau of Statistics and Australian Institute of Health and Welfare. ISSN 1441–2004 Commonwealth of Australia.

Sells DJ, Rowe M, Fisk D, Davidson L (2003) Violent victimization of persons with co-occurring psychiatric and substance use disorders. *Psychiatric Services* 54: 1253–1257.

Senate Select Committee on Mental Health (2006) A National Approach to Mental Health from Crisis to Community: First Report March 2006 ISBN 0 642 71636 6 Commonwealth of Australia.

Szirom T, King D, Desmond K (2004) *Barriers to Service Provision for Young People with Presenting Substance Misuse and Mental Health Problems. Success Works*. Canberra: NYARS National Youth Affairs Research Scheme.

Teeson M, Hall W, Lynskey M, Degenhardt L (2000) Alcohol and drug use disorders in Australia: Implications of the National Survey of Mental Health and Wellbeing. *Australian and New Zealand Journal of Psychiatry* 34: 206–213.

Victorian Government (2007) *Dual Diagnosis: Key Directions and Priorities for Service Development*. Melbourne: Victorian Government Department of Human Services.

Vos T, Barker B, Stanley L, Lopez A (2007) *The Burden of Disease and Injury in Aboriginal and Torres Strait Islander Peoples, 2003*. Brisbane: School of Population Health.

Wallace C, Mullen P, Burgess P (2004) Criminal offending in schizophrenia over a 25-year period marked by deinstitutionalization and increasing prevalence of comorbid substance use disorders. *American Journal of Psychiatry* 161: 716–727.

Chapter 20

Dual Diagnosis – Europe

Jane Salvage and Rob Keukens

Introduction

This chapter explores the social context, prevalence and treatment of problems related to dual diagnosis in the countries of Eastern Europe. It paints a picture of the region's historical and societal background; sets out basic epidemiological information; considers the rate and impact of mental illness and alcohol and substance abuse; reviews what services are available for people with dual diagnosis; outlines the barriers to progress and makes recommendations for improvements. The chapter draws on an extensive literature search as well as the authors' wide personal experience of working with mental health reformers in policy, education and service delivery in most countries in the region.

Just as it is impossible to give a single image of Western European practice, with its countless contradictions and local insights, a truly balanced image of developments is only possible through individual discussion of each of the 23 Eastern European countries; the overall situation can only be sketched in broad outlines. Nevertheless, despite the growing diversity of these countries and the paths they are taking, there is still remarkable homogeneity owing to the durability of their communist legacy. It remains possible to make some meaningful generalisations because mental health care is just one of many areas that have changed relatively little – shamefully little – in the two decades since the collapse of the Soviet Union.

The historical and social context

The term 'Eastern Europe', in the loose sense in which it is still widely used in many Western countries, refers to the former 'Eastern bloc' of countries behind the Iron Curtain that lay within the Soviet Union and its sphere of influence: a region with a common political history rather than geographical or cultural coherence. Following the collapse of the Soviet Union in 1989, its 15 republics gained independence and Czechoslovakia and the former Yugoslavia split into different countries while Germany was reunified. With more than 350 million people, the region covers a large swathe of the globe, from Central Europe to the far eastern shores of the Russian Federation, and from the Arctic north to the Caucasus and Central Asia in the south.

The old Communist rulers aimed to conceal and suppress internal differences and helped to create an undifferentiated image of Eastern Europe. This image does not do justice to the region's growing social and cultural diversity, encompassing modern democracies like the Czech Republic and Hungary that are now in the European Union, backward dictatorships like Turkmenistan and Uzbekistan, and other countries struggling somewhere in between to create a new identity and sense of direction. However, for nearly 20 years all these countries have been dealing with the impact of internal and external pressures for transition to more liberal ideologies, market-oriented economics and the slow development of civil society. This series of revolutions continues to have a huge impact, for both better and worse, on the health and psychosocial welfare of most of their populations.

The collapse of the Soviet Union brought many countries to the brink of chaos and dragged social and health structures down with it. Civil war, internal conflict, massive poverty, unemployment and migration were just some of the consequences of system breakdown and the forced march towards capitalism. The economic and social consequences were of varying profile and intensity. Millions of people fell below the poverty line and remain there, in capital cities now overrun by western tourists as well as forgotten corners of the former Yugoslavia, the Russian Federation, Central Asia and the Caucasus.

There is a strong, well-documented relationship between poverty and social deprivation, often accompanied by alcohol misuse and poor mental health (Perkins & Repper 2003). Worldwide, mental disorder is more common among people who are socially deprived, whether through the impact of poverty that predisposes to mental illness or the downward drift of mentally ill people and their families into poverty. Poverty and mental health interact in highly damaging ways and harm individuals, families, communities and entire societies. Lack of work and income usually lowers self-esteem, leading to a greater risk of depression and anxiety disorders, substance misuse, suicide and many physical illnesses. Suffering the double stigma of mental illness and poverty, some people seek money through crime or sex work, or follow health-damaging pursuits (such as unprotected sex and abuse of alcohol and drugs) in the search of temporary relief from their symptoms. Many end up in prison, where they are exposed to more health risks and their hopes of future employment vanish.

This scenario is clearly seen in Eastern Europe, where rapid economic and social changes have been accompanied by a decline in mental and physical health and a sharp increase in the incidence of substance abuse, prostitution, human immunodeficiency virus (HIV) and other sexually transmitted infections. As noted by Hamers and Downs (2003), these rapidly declining socio-economic conditions and increasing inequity have brought 'a sense of despair and hopelessness that is fertile ground for HIV transmission through increased risk behaviour including prostitution and drug use. A struggling economy means fewer resources for prevention and care'.

Average life expectancy has fallen and diseases previously controlled through primary health care and immunisation are rising again (Tomov *et al.* 2007), accompanied by the rapid spread of HIV/acquired immunodeficiency syndrome (AIDS). The average Russian man will die at 58 from the effects of a combination of poor nutrition, smoking and binge drinking. Mental illness rates are soaring, for example, suicide rates are extremely high, especially among men, with the incidence three times greater than in Western Europe (WHO 2001). Nine of the 10 countries with the highest suicide rates belong to the former Eastern bloc (Varnik 2002).

The factors that help protect people against mental illness and substance abuse, such as self-esteem, social cohesion and a sense of identity, have been undermined, as reflected in high levels of violence, divorce and suicide. Social safety nets for the poor and the ill are full of holes or have disintegrated. Many of the most economically active and skilled young workers are migrating, reducing family income. Meanwhile, social and health problems not only exacerbate the problems of dual diagnosis but also undermine the means of tackling them.

Elements of dual diagnosis in the region

Many people in the region suffer temporarily or on a long term from both a psychiatric condition and problems with substance use. The number of people in Russia referred to mental health clinics rose by over 14% between 1990 and 2000, primarily attributable to an increase in non-psychotic disorders and changing socio-economic changes (Neufeldt *et al.* 2002). In view of the dramatic rises in alcohol and drug consumption, it is highly likely that the number of people with a dual diagnosis has also increased substantially. All the determinants of dual diagnosis are gaining a stronger hold in many parts of Eastern Europe today. Below we look briefly at each in turn, and consider their lethal relationship with the rapid spread of HIV infection.

Alcohol

The European Union is the heaviest drinking region of the world, with an average annual alcohol consumption per capita (over 15 years old) of 11 litres

(Anderson & Baumberg 2006). Northern Europe and Eastern Europe have the highest health risks in relation to drinking patterns, especially binge drinking (WHO 2004). There are considerable variations: countries in south-eastern Europe with a more Mediterranean lifestyle, such as Bulgaria and Romania, have an estimated consumption around the European average, while the Czech Republic, Hungary, Latvia, Lithuania and Slovakia have the highest rates. The yearly average consumption per capita in the Russian Federation is estimated at 15 litres. In some areas the prevalence of alcohol use disorders is over 5% of the highest in the world. A third of the deaths in the Russian Federation are said to be alcohol-related, rising to 43% among men aged 25–54 (Leon *et al.* 2007). There has been an increase in newborns with fetal alcohol syndrome.

Eastern European countries have long been known to have an impressive drinking culture, and a large intake is not considered problematic in contrast with drug use which is often demonised. There seems to be an explosive increase in consumption with heavy use of moonshine and other home-made substances; people drink everything that alters the mind, from antifreeze to varnish. The characters in Venedikt Erofeev's 1994 novel *Moscow to the End of the Line* drink a lethal cocktail called 'Tears of a Komsomol Girl', containing eau-de-cologne, lemon soda, nail polish, lavender and mouthwash. Young people are at particular risk of becoming addicted (WHO 2003). Most countries have no coherent policy to reduce alcohol consumption, for example, by random breath testing, implementing a minimum drinking age, raising taxation or limiting sales opportunities.

Other psychoactive substances

Drug use was very heavily penalised by the state under Communism, but government controls have relaxed or even disappeared. Meanwhile the import and transit of illegal drugs via former Soviet republics such as Tajikistan has become much easier; the diversification of trafficking routes through Central Asia and Eastern Europe brings relatively cheap heroin to the streets of former Soviet cities. It is difficult to quantify this consumption, because most users are unlikely to be registered, and official data are often misleading. The actual number of drug users everywhere is probably much greater than official statistics suggest.

The use of illicit drugs is growing fast, with injecting drug use playing an increasing role in transmitting HIV and hepatitis. The newly independent states of the former Soviet Union all show alarming increases in the number of people using drugs. In Kyrgyzstan, an estimated 2% of the adult population injects drugs (UNAIDS 2004), while in Georgia 70% of those registered with HIV have injected drugs. In 2004, 343,000 drug-dependent people were officially registered in the Russian Federation, but the real number may be ten times greater (Dolzhankaya *et al.* 2006). The use of cannabis in the Eastern European countries of the EU is relatively limited, although its popularity is rising and there are regional differences (EMCDDA 2006). The prevalence among 15- to 34-year-olds is 4% in Bulgaria, 5% in Lithuania and 8% in Latvia, compared to 12% in the Netherlands and 20% in the frontrunner Spain. The lifetime prevalence of cannabis use among young people in the Russian Federation and the Ukraine is estimated at 20%, while the use of other types of drugs including home-made substances like Jeff, a stimulant, or Cherniashka, an opiate, is estimated at more than 4%. The use of inhalants among young people in Russia and the Ukraine has a lifetime prevalence of approximately 10%. The prevalence of cocaine use among people older than 15 is less than 0.5% in the Baltic States and Bulgaria, compared with 2% in England.

Human immunodeficiency virus/acquired immunodeficiency syndrome

One of the consequences of the increasing use of psychoactive substances in the region, particularly heroin, is the rapid and uncontrolled spread of HIV/AIDS. An estimated 1.7 million people in the region are living with HIV, with 90% in the Russian Federation and the Ukraine. This catastrophic figure represents an almost 20-fold increase in less than a decade, while the infection rate in countries like Georgia and Moldova has doubled in 5 years (UNAIDS 2006). Injecting drug use is the main route of transmission in all countries, through the use of non-sterile injecting equipment, but the patterns of the epidemic are changing in several countries. Sexually transmitted HIV cases comprise a growing share of new diagnoses – 45% in Moldova in 2004, for example (EuroHIV 2005). While most of those currently seropositive are men, increasing numbers of women are being infected – many by male partners who become infected while injecting drugs. More children are being born to HIV-positive mothers, making prevention of mother-to-child transmission a priority (UNAIDS 2005).

This grim development raises the issue of a growth in 'triple diagnosis' of mental illness, substance abuse and HIV/AIDS (Box 20.1). The mental health problems associated with HIV are well documented: mental illness and addictions increase vulnerability to infection, while being diagnosed with HIV/AIDS has profound effects on mental well-being through the associated stigma and discrimination as well as through the progression of the disease itself. Around three-quarters of people with HIV/AIDS will have at least one psychiatric disorder in their lifetime (Baingana *et al.* 2005). HIV-positive, injecting drug users have higher levels of cognitive impairment, mood disorders, suicide attempts and completed suicides compared to HIV-positive people who are not injecting drug users (Kalichman 1995). The poor economic and social conditions that underpin burgeoning HIV infection rates also underpin proliferating mental health problems. Furthermore, mental health problems, drug and alcohol misuse and learning difficulties can influence behaviour in ways that lead to greater risk of HIV infection. Populations that are particularly at risk already have higher rates of mental illness, including injecting drug users, sex workers, refugees and migrants and prisoners.

Box 20.1   The lethal cocktail of triple diagnosis

- Untreated mental illness and addiction > risk-taking behaviour > spread of HIV
- Untreated mental illness and addiction > lower adherence to antiretroviral therapy (ART) > spread of HIV and poorer prognosis
- ART > side effects damaging to mental health
- AIDS > brain impairment and other impacts on mental functioning
- Untreated mental illness and addiction > poorer quality of life for people living with HIV/AIDS (PLHA)
- Untreated mental illness and addiction > greater stress on carers and families
- Lack of social and community support > social exclusion > more illness, poverty and despair.

Care and treatment responses

People with these coexisting problems face multiple types of stigma relating to their HIV status, mental illness and substance misuse, and may have additional difficulties in accessing and adhering to treatment and care, as the case study of Elena suggests. Health and social care systems in the region cannot at present cope with the enormous challenge. Except for a few private services accessible only to the wealthy, they are mostly underfunded and poorly equipped and supplied and lack professionals with adequate training, knowledge and expertise. Modern medicines are often hard to obtain. Even when good mental health services are available, which are very unusual, poor people often cannot afford to travel to clinics, pay the professionals (officially or under the table) or buy medications.

CASE STUDY 1: ELENA
This case study is based on a true story from Kyrgyzstan, but names and some details have been changed.

Elena, 51, is a single mother with a son aged 13. Four years ago she discovered that she was HIV-positive while having hospital treatment and taking the blood test. Her first reactions were suicidal thoughts – she felt there was no point in going on living – followed by fears for her son's future. She has no relatives who could support her and her son. She became addicted to alcohol before she learned of her HIV status, attributing this to her constant feelings of depression: no desire to live, no energy and no willpower. She then lost her job. She does not want to be treated at an AIDS centre because the first time she attended, the professional she saw was unsupportive and seemed uncaring. She has not tried to find other AIDS professionals to support her because she feared meeting this type of reaction again, and she did not believe that anyone could help her anyway. Finally, with the support and encouragement of a doctor at the centre where she is treated for her addiction, she accepted a referral to the hospital responsible for ART. She is now waiting for her treatment, which she hopes will start soon.

People of all ages with developmental, mental or behavioural problems are isolated from others and from society, sometimes placed in long-stay health or social care institutions for years and exposed to violation of their rights. If their families are unable or unwilling to care for them they are sent to asylums or residential homes, often far from home. They have little or no say in their treatment or how long they stay there, and no support if they are ill-treated. If they come out, there are usually no community-based services to help them maintain their treatment, let alone reintegrate into society or find work. Families trying to cope with the many social and economic pressures of having a relative with schizophrenia or dementia may come to believe that putting them in an institution is the only option, or even the best one.

The number of adequately trained mental health workers (whether psychiatrists, psychologists, nurses or social workers) is insufficient to meet the needs. Their training, where it exists, is usually out of date and there is very little continuing education. Professionals in other parts of the health system have little expertise in mental health. Mental health services in Eastern Europe grew in the shadows of Moscow's Serbsky Institute, which remains Russia's leading hospital and academic centre for forensic psychiatry. When it worked as an arm of the KGB or secret police, the institute devised implausible diagnoses such as 'sluggish schizophrenia' as a pretext for confining dissidents to mental hospitals. Its psychiatrists employed dubious scientific methods to interpret human behaviour in a biomedical way that categorised anything differing from a rigidly defined norm as organically deviant, curable only by medication and institutionalisation.

This pseudoscience lingers on, with patients' problems still often classified according to discredited beliefs and terminology, while the predominance of a single school or view limits the spectrum of available treatment modalities. Many proven interventions are ruled out: for example, methadone substitution is prohibited by the Russian government, which focuses on abstinence. Health professional responses are strongly determined by the reductionist medical bias of their training, and their lack of knowledge of addiction and its social-psychological dimensions, harm reduction and primary health care interventions. Professionals are often fatalistic and describe patients in terms of their shortcomings, bringing few positive expectations and making negative moral judgments (as shown in both case studies). Professionals in addiction clinics mostly focus on detoxification with the goal of complete abstinence, although their expectations of success are very low. Non-mental-health professionals do not see diagnostics and screening of addiction problems as their responsibility. Repressive and disapproving attitudes to drug-dependent people mean that every user, including those who maintain their usage in a socially acceptable manner, is labelled an 'addict' or 'problem case'.

The region hosts a vast and rich range of cultures, each with its own assumptions about mental illness and its own ways of dealing with it. Some aspects of this are positive and caring, but others are not. People who are mentally ill are deemed antisocial and threatening, and most health workers reinforce this stigmatisation. People with a dual diagnosis are doubly or triply stigmatised and few services tackle their needs. Access to treatment of any kind is rare to non-existent for HIV-positive injecting drug users. All these problems are even more evident in services (or lack of them) for people in settings such as prisons, where conditions are generally appalling, general health services very inadequate and mental health services absent. Treatment regimes in existing services are of a general nature and focus on detoxification and abstinence. The notion that these people are in need of integrated, tailor-made services is slowly gaining ground, but has not yet led to solid government initiatives. Assessing substance misuse and establishing links with drug and alcohol dependency agencies are important in the medical and psychological management of HIV infection, but there is little or no cooperation between psychiatric institutions, primary health care, social services and voluntary organisations, and only a few self-help and user groups have started up.

Problems and solutions

This brief review of the problems associated with dual diagnosis highlights the importance of tackling them, for individuals, communities and countries, and also their great complexity. They are by nature very difficult to solve, while the people who experience them may be hard to reach and help. Health and social care systems in the region cannot at present cope with the challenges, and there are fears that rapid socio-economic changes mean things could get worse before they get better (Knapp *et al.* 2007).

Bleak as this picture is, there are some bright spots. One is the huge decline in the political abuse of psychiatry, thanks to the vigilance of dedicated human rights activists. Another is the growing determination among citizens – including people with mental health problems, their families and reform-minded professionals – to transform mental health services and social attitudes. A range of projects, often with external support and funding, is reconfiguring services, letting fresh air and fresh ideas into closed institutions, developing networks, rewriting repressive legislation, updating training curricula and starting to put the person with mental health needs at the centre of planning and service delivery.

Another positive sign is the growing interest in mental health issues worldwide. WHO devoted its 2001 world health report to mental illness, and most Eastern European governments signed up the declaration and action plan agreed upon at the WHO European ministerial conference on mental health (WHO 2005). The EU is developing new mental health policies and networks and beginning to support mental health projects. Further east, financial support for such work is thin and increasingly hard to obtain. Sadly, mental health development is itself stigmatised by most donors who have invested little despite the scale of the problems. Progress is painfully slow.

A few special initiatives have been initiated via foreign aid programmes. For example, the Minnesota model is being used on a small scale in different countries – a comprehensive, interdisciplinary abstinence-based treatment approach based on the Alcoholics Anonymous 12-step model. Counselling techniques such as motivational interviewing are also being tried, and harm reduction interventions such as needle exchange programmes in Albania, Georgia, Romania, the Russian Federation and elsewhere. The Mental Health and HIV/AIDS (MAIDS) project of the Global Initiative on Psychiatry is a unique multinational project where the problem of dual/triple diagnosis has a prominent role (Global Initiative on Psychiatry 2006).

As in all other areas of development, mental health reform will succeed only if it is owned by and led by the people themselves. National governments have been slow to act on the scandalous treatment of mentally ill people, and in most countries reform efforts have started not with the policy makers but with a few brave service users, families and professionals. Helped by the slow growth of civil society, non-governmental organisations have been founded to tackle mental health needs: many were started by the mothers and wives of people with mental illness or learning disabilities, to provide previously non-existent support services such as day centres, clubs and self-help groups. There are far too few of them and they often find themselves in conflict with uninterested or even hostile policy makers and public service leaders. The Russian Federation's xenophobic restrictions on NGO activity are just one example. Yet NGOs like Bemoni in Georgia, Somato in Moldova, and Mental Health and Society in Kyrgyzstan provide inspiring examples of what can be achieved (see also Case study 2).

CASE STUDY 2: DANY

This case study is based on a true story from the Republic of Moldova, but names and some details have been changed.

Dany displayed the first signs of paranoid schizophrenia when he was 19. The crisis was manifested through vagrancy, refusing to eat, fearing he would be poisoned and thinking he had no place in his family home. At the age of 22 he was admitted to the psychiatric hospital for the fourth time, from the place where he had lived with other drug users. Dany was tested for HIV without being asked for his consent, because testing was compulsory for people from at-risk groups. He was found to be HIV-positive. His mother worked at the hospital as a nurse and, learning about his HIV status, rejected him. Neighbours and colleagues did the same. He is alone and lives on the street. The only help he gets is from a community mental health centre set up by a non-governmental organisation. The centre aims to help Dany achieve some stability in his life and cope with his diagnoses of schizophrenia and HIV.

One example of this empowering approach is the Cherkassy project in the Ukraine, which has introduced new approaches to the prevention of psychoactive substance abuse. Financed by the Dutch Ministry of Foreign Affairs, it resulted in the introduction of systematic education in secondary schools and summer camps, achieved through international training events; peer-to-peer prevention lessons among pupils, parents and school staff; distribution of manuals, leaflets, brochures and films; development of a regional network of prevention workers; small community prevention projects; performances of social/psychological prevention theatre and the development of a network. The 3-year project was followed up with development of a comprehensive programme on psychoactive substance prevention education.

Another example is a series of conferences on community-based substance abuse treatment programmes that took place in 2003–2004 with the network of young reformers in substance abuse. About 30 professionals with backgrounds in mental health, psychiatry and substance abuse care and treatment participated in two training seminars. Apart from the group dynamic dimensions such as networking, cooperation, interaction and information exchange, the participants strengthened their skills in drug policy; drug service development; community orientation; and care, treatment and prevention interventions.

Reform will require many more funded initiatives like these to foster significant shifts in attitude and culture, greater knowledge, full collaboration between services, multidisciplinary teamwork and user involvement – all the ingredients necessary to create a modern, ethical, client-oriented care system. Just as importantly, the powerful negative influence of the breakdown of social networks, communities and families throughout the region must be tackled in a revival of the community spirit damaged or destroyed by poverty, civil war, migration, corruption and the loss of traditional attitudes, practices and cultures that helped people to cope with hardship.

Conclusion

The human toll of change in Eastern Europe is huge, but so far no government or international agency has risen fully to the task of visualising a realistic future and way ahead for health systems and providing the necessary political will and resources to make change happen. This persistent failure of governance is predicated on deeply instilled dependency, corruption and indifference to and attacks on individuality, which was the hallmark of the previous regimes. The backdrop of globalisation adds further frustrations to those arising from the need to replace passivity with social participation – faced by every single citizen. The challenge is no longer to find a dependable employer or patron, but to reshape dependency needs by adopting an entrepreneurial stance, that is, a psychic organization enabling interdependence. Yet a huge proportion of the region's ageing population is deprived of the chance to make this transition.

Tackling the problems of dual diagnosis in Eastern Europe therefore requires a major effort. Governments are reluctant to take responsibility to make good policy and to allocate adequate resources to mental health and services for people with drug and alcohol problems. Their countries are mostly economically insecure, and some are politically unstable, especially outside the EU. Drastic, structured measures are required rather than the current tendency for crisis management through ad hoc policy measures and short-term programmes. The issue of dual diagnosis will have to be placed on the agenda, not least because young people and thus the future social capital of the region are at stake. Intersectoral cooperation will have to help remove the artificial divisions between narcology, mental health and primary health care and prevention. Human resources development is vital, with a focus on evidence-based promotion of expertise. The strengthening of client and family movements is necessary to fight stigma and strengthen legal rights.

Developments in this specific area will depend on progress in health care in general. We make some recommendations in Box 20.2. Mental health has never been a priority: the tremendous task facing Eastern Europe requires huge efforts now and for the foreseeable future. Initiatives to create civil society, promote social inclusion and build capacity will all be crucial in tackling dual diagnosis, while the implications for policy and practice extend far beyond the traditional boundaries of health services.

Box 20.2   Recommendations for tackling dual diagnosis problems in Eastern Europe

- Assess awareness, expertise and training needs of health and social care services (state and non-governmental) that provide dual diagnosis care and treatment, as a foundation for developing programmes and strengthening referral networks.
- Provide training for primary and secondary health and social care staff in the recognition, prevention and treatment of dual diagnosis. People living with the problem should be involved in the planning and provision of training.
- Identify existing materials for training, education and self-help, and adapt and translate into local languages for local use, with development of new materials based on needs assessment.
- Expand services including counselling, psychosocial support groups, treatment of substance use, psychological and psychiatric assessment and treatment, self-help resources and social interventions such as occupational training.
- Strengthen community awareness by establishing partnerships and networking with a range of stakeholders in primary care, hospitals, prisons, community groups, schools, mental health user and carer groups, the media and policy makers.
- Address stigma and discrimination at policy and practice levels, including public education and awareness campaigns.

References

Anderson P, Baumberg B (2006) *Alcohol in Europe. A Public Health Perspective.* Cambridge: European Union/Institute of Alcohol Studies.

Baingana F, Thomas R, Comblain C (2005) *HIV/AIDS and Mental Health.* Health, Nutrition and Population Discussion Paper, World Bank. Free download from www.worldbank.org.

Dolzhankaya N, Bouzina T, Kozlov A, *et al.* (2006) Knowledge and attitudes of drug treatment professionals towards HIV prevention and care activities in the Russian Federation. *Heroin Addiction and Related Clinical Problems* 8: 23–25.

EuroHIV (2005) *HIV/AIDS Surveillance in Europe,* End-year report 2004, 2005 no 71 www.eurohiv.org/reports/report_71/pdf/report_eurohiv_71.pdf.

European Monitoring Centre for Drugs and Drug Addiction (2006) Annual Report. http://www.emcdda.europa.eu.

Global Initiative on Psychiatry (2006) *Double Stigma, Double Challenge: Mental Health and HIV/AIDS in Central and Eastern Europe and the Newly Independent States. Advocacy and Information Document.* Hilversum: GIP.

Hamers F, Downs A (2003) HIV in central and eastern Europe. *The Lancet* 361: 1035–1044.

Kalichman S (1995) *Understanding AIDS: A Guide for Mental Health Professionals*. Washington DC: American Psychological Association.

Knapp M, McDaid D, Mossalios E, Thornicroft G (2007) Mental health policy and practice across Europe: an overview. In Knapp M, McDaid D, Mossalios E, Thornicroft G (eds) *Mental Health Policy and Practice across Europe*. Milton Keynes, UK: Open University Press.

Leon D, Saburova L, Tomkins S, *et al.* (2007) Hazardous alcohol drinking and premature mortality in Russia: a population based case-control study. *The Lancet* 369: 2001–2009.

Neufeldt A, Toews J, Shklarov S, *et al.* (2002) Russian mental health system reform. In *Final Report, Community Rehabilitation and Disability Studies Programme*. Calgary, Canada: University of Calgary and Moscow Research Institute of Psychiatry.

Perkins R, Repper J (2003) *Social Inclusion and Recovery: A Model for Mental Health Practice*. Edinburgh: Elsevier Health Sciences.

Tomov T, Voren R, van Keukens R (2007) Mental health policy in former Eastern Bloc countries. In Knapp M, McDaid D, Mossalios E, Thornicroft G (eds). *Mental Health Policy and Practice across Europe*. Milton Keynes, UK: Open University Press.

UNAIDS (2004) *Report on the Global AIDS Epidemic*. Geneva, Switzerland: UNAIDS.

UNAIDS (2005) *Report on the Global AIDS Epidemic*. Geneva, Switzerland: UNAIDS.

UNAIDS (2006) *Fact Sheet: Eastern Europe and Central Asia*. Geneva, Switzerland: UNAIDS.

Varnik A (2002) *Depression and Mental Health in Estonia*. Geneva: WHO.

World Health Organization (2001) *Mental Health: New Understanding, New Hope*. World Health Report 2001. Geneva: WHO.

World Health Organization (2003) *Substance Abuse in Central and Eastern Europe. Summary of Baseline Assessment in Belarus and the Russian Federation*. Geneva: WHO.

World Health Organization (2004) *Global Status Report on Alcohol*. Geneva: WHO Department of Mental Health and Substance Abuse.

World Health Organization (2005) Mental health: facing the challenges, building solutions. In: *Declaration and Action Plan on Mental Health, European Ministerial Conference, Helsinki*. Copenhagen: WHO Regional Office for Europe.

Chapter 21

Commissioning Services for Users with Dual Diagnosis

Sharon Dennis

Introduction

The term dual diagnosis has been in use in mental health services for less than 15 years. Traditionally, mental health has followed the medical model in that practitioners focused on only one aspect of the service user's care, expecting other services or agencies to deal with the other issues. In the case of dual diagnosis, a recent policy document (DH 2002) acknowledges that mental health and substance misuse services have evolved separately and, at the time of the document's inception, few services existed to address the needs of those who had both substance and alcohol misuse issues in conjunction with a mental health problem.

The practice of compartmentalising a person's care has often meant that users fall between services and do not receive the care and treatment required that facilitates recovery. Small wonder then that there is a dearth of literature that specifically addresses the commissioning of dual diagnosis services.

This chapter draws on the development of commissioning in the United Kingdom's National Health Service (NHS) and considers the implications for dual diagnosis services.

Background

When the NHS was initiated in 1948, the Labour government was concerned that as health care had been available only for those with the ability to pay, the ongoing health of the population could not be systematically improved. The consequence of this was that the availability of sufficient numbers of healthy workers in post-war Britain could not be predicted. The government believed that after improving the health of the nation, they would be able to wind down the UK health service they had established. At that time the service consisted of hospital care, access to a network of general practitioners (GPs) and community care (Greengross *et al.* 1999).

Instead of becoming unnecessary, the NHS has become the world's third largest employer, as it has expanded the range and depth of services available. Services were usually developed as a result of local clinical interest rather than any systematic grand plan. The Department of Health (DH) – which has responsibility for national strategies – placed responsibility for overviewing local services with regional health authorities who exerted some control over service development in an attempt to ensure equity of availability and to promote research. Nevertheless, the term 'post code lottery', which means that access to treatment is not entirely based on need but on decisions made by local health leaders who have set their own priorities, has become an accepted reality within the UK health care.

A major change came in 1989 when an 'internal market' was introduced by the DH in the document *Working for Patients* (DH 1989) which was a first attempt to introduce a business model to the NHS. For the first time, a clear differentiation between those who provide health services and those who purchase or commission them was made. In addition, standards for services to meet were also set, and reward for those who were deemed to meet those standards were made available.

At the time of writing, Foundation status is the accolade set for NHS trusts to achieve. Many NHS mental health and drug service providers are pursuing this goal and the carrot for this achievement is less control from the central government. The theory is that organizations that are consistently unable to achieve the standards set would ultimately cease to exist as they would be taken over by those able to perform.

The history of commissioning

The NHS has undergone many reorganizations and the introduction of primary care trusts (PCTs) from 2001 onwards was a turning point in the development of commissioning. A primary care trust at that time had the responsibility for both delivering services (being a provider) and ensuring that an appropriate range of services was available for a defined population by contracting for these (purchasing). In terms of delivery, GPs are key to local health care (see Chapter 20). These doctors offer both direct treatment and access to a range of services such as district nurses, health visitors, physiotherapy and others. In addition, GPs are the gateway to specialist treatment in hospital.

Commissioning involves purchasing, monitoring and manipulation. It has been defined as follows: 'Commissioning is the strategic planning and resource allocation function of the NHS, mostly done by PCTs. It involves buying in services from a range of health service providers . . . . to meet the health needs of local people, and monitoring how well they are being delivered' (NHS Alliance 2006). Manipulation comes into play as commissioners set criteria for services and ask providers to bid against those criteria for the contract. This stimulates competition and should improve value for money and drive standards up.

In the early 2000s, the responsibility for commissioning was given to new organisations with staff who had no experience in this role. When PCTs first took on this function there would have been no written contracts or service standards that they could use as a baseline. Additionally, there is no agreed standard for the background experience of qualification of commissioners. It is not unusual for these crucial staff not to have any experience of the services they are commissioning.

On a global level, each PCT is allocated funds by the DH, and the DH has constructed a complex matrix of responsibility for commissioning. This is currently on four different levels – national, specialist, local and practice based. Around 80% of the total NHS budget is devolved to PCTs while the rest includes an allocation for services which are commissioned at either Strategic Health Authority or national levels for a given population. Overall mental health accounts for approximately 12% of the total NHS budget; as such, it was a low priority for commissioners in the early days as they got to grips with their roles.

PCTs struggled with being both providers and commissioners of care, effectively buying some of the health care the population required from themselves. However, in 2005, the policy document *Commissioning a Patient Led NHS* indicated that PCTs could become 'commissioning-only' organisations and divest themselves of their hitherto provider functions. While many PCTs continued to provide as well as commission services, many set up systems that divided these two functions within the organisation in order to demonstrate their impartiality in choosing providers. Furthermore, in 2005/2006 the number of PCTs was dramatically reduced with a number of mergers taking place. The ongoing changes within PCTs detracted commissioners from being able to concentrate their efforts on relatively small services like dual diagnosis.

Up until this point PCTs had held more of a contracting function, that is, choosing their provision from what was already available, rather than that of true commissioners who develop services. The DH describes world class commissioning as including collaborating with clinicians, the public and partners, and stimulating and developing the local health service. The concept of world class commissioning was clearly influenced by the Health Policy Forum (Smith *et al.* 2006) research which described effective commissioning as having four main components: the identification of need and demand, the shaping of markets, holding the market to account and holding commissioners to account (Modernisation Agency 2005).

The Health Policy Forum (Smith *et al.* 2006) policy document outlines a crucial element of accountability – the need for commissioners themselves to be monitored in terms of performance. Examples such as engaging the public and governance are described.

In reality, at the time of writing, these policies have not made a major impact on service users or service development.

Implications for commissioning dual diagnosis services

Substance misuse services had traditionally been provided under the umbrella of mental health services but often with a range of funding streams. With the funding also comes specific guidance on how that money is spent. More recently service provision has become even more complex with providers within the charity and independent sector also becoming significant players as regards service provision. In addition, service users presenting with a dual diagnosis often found that their care has been fragmented at best and inadequate at worst with mental health services not addressing their substance misuse issues and, vice versa.

World class commissioning builds on the document published in early 2007, *Commissioning Framework for Health and Well-being* (DH 2007a), which outlines plans for strengthening interventions for prevention as well as the provision of health care and capitalising on the use of local information about the population to drive future commissioning decisions. In terms of mental health particularly, health commissioning is significant but not the entire story. The commissioning of social care is equally important as both health and social interventions are usually required in order to provide a comprehensive care package. In order to cover both social and health care commissioning, many PCTs and local authorities have agreed to combine their resources to establish joint commissioning roles and teams.

In addition to commissioning and providing social care, local authorities have a responsibility under the Health and Social Care Act 2001 to monitor local health services via overview and scrutiny committees (OSCs). Ultimately the OSC can refer matters to the Secretary of State for Health, but due to the OSC's wide remit the ongoing monitoring of mental health services including dual diagnosis is the responsibility of the Local implementation Team (LIT). The LITs were set up after the introduction of the National Service Framework; this combination of service users, carers, commissioners and providers monitors the progress in achieving nationally set standards. The local Drug Action Team (DAT) provides a similar role for substance misuse teams. Clearly, the two need to work closely to ensure service users' needs to be met; however, the LIT has been given the lead role for dual diagnosis.

The aspirational document, *World Class Commissioning: Vision* (DH 2007b) introduces the strap-line 'adding life to years and years to life'. This objective is in keeping with the national target regarding the reduction of drug-related deaths (National Treatment Agency 1999). The world class commissioning vision includes standards for PCTs. The vision includes three objectives: better health and well-being for all, better care for all and better value for all. The policy therefore covers public health and reducing inequalities, improving standards of care and demonstrating the effective management of resources.

For specific guidance on dual diagnosis, the *Mental Health Policy Implementation Guide: Dual Diagnosis Good Practice Guide* (DH 2002) is clear in stating that services should be 'mainstreamed' and therefore available within general mental health services. Any commissioner will additionally need to be mindful of the matrix within the document which describes an individual on two – the axis of substance misuse and the mental health problem and rating the severity of each from low to high. Services that are commissioned should offer treatment that clearly relates to the severity of the presenting symptoms.

Commissioners must therefore be aware of this spectrum – and the volume of local need – and have systems in place for both placing contracts for care across this range and monitoring the provision. While the policy documents on commissioning encourage the purchase of services from a range of providers, most commissions are within the NHS. Indeed, NHS contracting and the need to have a stable health economy – the latter is overseen by the Strategic Health Authority – mitigate against major and/or rapid changes in previous commissioning arrangements. Furthermore, the DH has introduced a system of national tariffs for various treatments in order for incentive providers to demonstrate value for money. In conjunction with tariffs a system called payment by results has introduced a cost and volume approach to commissioning. This system necessitates commissioners predicting the number of treatments required and guarantees payment for same; this led to situations where providers could no longer offer a treatment within a financial year when the money ran out.

As the years have gone on more sophisticated arrangements have been agreed in order to avoid this disastrous scenario. These include contracting over a 3-year period and agreeing a rate of payment for treatments carried out over the originally agreed figure.

At the time of writing, practice-based commissioning is voluntary and has not been fully embedded; however some PCTs have set up systems to facilitate the commissioning of services by local clinicians. This has proved more problematic for the commissioning of mental health services, as national tariffs have not yet been set. In addition, the small numbers of particular treatments that may be required may lead to difficulties in predicting future need and therefore the cost effective use of resources. In order to ensure sufficient numbers of places are commissioned, GP practices may commission as a 'cluster' or, commissioning organisations jointly commission as a consortium.

The development of services for this client group is a key priority. Integrated care appears to confer superior outcomes over serial or parallel treatment although further well-designed research is required. Integrated treatment in the United Kingdom can be delivered by existing mental health services following training. With close liaison and support from substance misuse services, the choice of approach should be informed by local factors with input from all major stakeholders, and must deliver the objectives set out as follows:

- All mental health provider agencies must designate a lead-clinician for dual diagnosis issues.
- All health and social care economies must set up a project team to lead on implementing this guide.
- All health and social care economies must designate a lead commissioner.
- The team must agree on a local focused definition, care pathways and other required protocols/agreements.
- A two-tiered training strategy must deliver basic training across all staff in relevant services and advanced training.
- Supervision for particular staff must be formulated and implemented.

(From *Mental Health Policy Implementation Guide: Dual Diagnosis Good Practice Guide* 2002.)

Conclusion

The needs of dual diagnosis service users are complex and the challenges for commissioning of dual diagnosis services are many. Effective commissioning relies on commissioners who understand the needs of service users and can craft solutions from the range of funding streams while ensuring that mainstream mental health takes the lead on provision. In addition, LITs and other forums for reviewing local service provision need to keep the development and outcomes of services for this group high on their agenda.

This is reflected in the 5-year review of the implementation of the National Service Framework for Mental Health (Appleby 2004) which specifically noted that addressing the needs of service users with dual diagnosis remains a major priority and, there is still a long way to go for both commissioners and providers in ensuring that appropriate services are available.

References

Appleby L (2004) *National Service Framework for Mental Health – Five Years on London*. London: Department of Health.

Department of Health (1989) *Working for Patients*. London: HMSO.

Department of Health (2002) *Mental Health Policy Implementation Guide: Dual Diagnosis Good Practice Guide*. London: HMSO.

Department of Health (2007a) *Commissioning Framework for Health and Well-being*. London: HMSO.

Department of Health (2007b) *World Class Commissioning: Vision*. London: DH.

Greengross P, Grant K, Collini E (1999) *The History and Development of the UK National Health Service 1948–1999*. London: DFID Health Systems Resource Centre.

Modernisation Agency (2005) *The Commissioning Friend for Mental Health Services*. Leeds: NIMHE.

National Treatment Agency (1999) *Commissioning Services to Reduce Drug-Related Deaths*. London: DH.

NHS Alliance (2006) Crunch Time for NHS Commissioning (Press Release) London.

Smith JA, Lewis R, Harrison T (2006) *Making Commissioning Effective in the Reformed NHS in England*. London: The Health Policy Forum.

Chapter 22

Practice, Research and Education Development

Kevin Gournay

Introduction

Some 12 years ago, the writer of this chapter and one of the editors of this book (TS) made a range of arguments for saying that dual diagnosis should be seen as a major priority for mental health nursing (Gournay *et al.* 1997). Although, as this book testifies, there has, since that time, been a wide range of initiatives launched to confront the problem, it remains – in the writer's view – debatable whether real progress has been made in dealing with what is arguably the most formidable challenge to today's mental health services. As a preface to considering developments in practice, research and education, one needs to put the issue of dual diagnosis into a much wider societal context. In the United Kingdom there is now unrestricted access to alcohol on a 24-hour basis, cannabis has been downgraded in its classification and there is wide acceptance that these drugs are not only easily accessible to all, but also relatively much cheaper in price. Drugs, such as cocaine, which were once seen as exclusive drugs consumed by the very rich, are now available to all, including schoolchildren, and we have reached a situation where getting high on Class A drugs is a much cheaper option to augment an evening out than buying a few bottles of lager. One might argue that the wider changes in society serve to minimise the impact of anything that we can do in mental health services to deal with the problem.

Research

Before considering the research findings, it is important to make a few preliminary comments regarding what research needs to be done and the practical difficulties of carrying out research that will make a real contribution to dealing with the problem.

What research needs to be done?

First, we need to understand much more about the nature of dual diagnosis and there is still a need to deal with the conundrum of what causes what. This is not a new question. Indeed, Quitkin *et al.* (1972) estimated that 5–10% of people with agoraphobia abused drugs and alcohol and, then Mullaney and Trippett (1979) found that many people entering an alcohol treatment facility had phobic anxiety and that the majority of those people had a phobic anxiety before the onset of their excessive use of alcohol.

Researchers are still attempting to tease out what comes first, the mental illness or the drug use (Barnett *et al.* 2007). However, the research questions regarding causation are made even more difficult to investigate because of the wide variation in substances used and the fact that the substances used may vary over time and people may use single substances or substances in combination.

With regard to the problems of carrying out research studies on interventions, there are substantial difficulties. To begin, the nature of the problem varies because the populations that need to be studied will have not only a range of different substances used but also a range of psychiatric diagnoses. The nature of the population also makes recruitment into research studies difficult and, arguably, the people who most need to be studied are those least likely to enter research programmes. Once people have entered research programmes, the drop-out rates are also very high and therefore the group studied at follow-up may be atypical of the population. While there is now substantial research into the problem and interventions used, there is also the further difficulty of lack of agreement between research authorities on the outcome measures to be used, thus making consideration of results difficult.

Research in dual diagnosis has considered two central areas, the first being the nature of the problem and the impact on the person and the mental health service and the second being the interventions.

With regard to research on the nature of the problem and consequences, there is a generally accepted figure of 50% of people with a severe mental illness using illicit drugs and/or alcohol at hazardous levels (Cleary *et al.* 2008). In turn, people with dual diagnosis are much more likely to be admitted to hospital, to receive prison sentences or to commit violent crime than the general population (Frischer *et al.* 2004). It is also clear that people with dual diagnosis have higher rates of suicide and a wide range of physical illnesses, including hepatitis and HIV (Cleary *et al.* 2008). With regard to interventions, for a definitive overview of all psychosocial interventions, the reader is referred to the excellent Cochrane Systematic Review by Cleary *et al.* (2008). This review considered 25 randomised controlled trials and the authors concluded that there was

> *No compelling evidence to support any one psychosocial treatment over another to reduce substance use (or improve mental state) by people with serious mental illnesses.*

The authors drew attention to the various difficulties involved in carrying out research and called for improvements in research approaches. Included in the analysis of research findings was a wide range of interventions, from cognitive behaviour therapy and motivational interviewing, to 12-step approaches, such as used by Narcotics and Alcoholics Anonymous. These treatments under scrutiny came in different formats, sometimes as a one-off treatment and some delivered as part of an integrated programme. The authors also concluded that none of the treatments demonstrated that specific psychosocial interventions for people with severe mental illness and substance misuse were any better than treatment as usual. Consideration of these trials also reveals that many of the interventions delivered were carried out by people with very high levels of training. The report pointed out that it is difficult to see how such studies would generalise to the 'real world'. Indeed, this is a problem with many studies of psychological intervention.

One of the ongoing debates in dual diagnosis services is whether interventions for dual diagnosis should be delivered by specialist teams of workers, or integrated across the entire community mental health team. The latter approach is of course the current UK government policy. A recent study conducted in an inner city area of London demonstrated that mainstreaming dual diagnosis interventions did not seem to add to beneficial outcomes (Johnson *et al.* 2007). Thus in respect of research, one could conclude that, while the last decade has seen a great increase in research, we have learned little about what may be truly effective. We also are beginning to realise that the application of research in this area is compromised by two issues. The first is that of developing a methodologically sound protocol, with attention given to sampling, design and outcome measures, and second the problem of developing a research programme that produces results that are of benefit to real world services. In many respects, these two objectives are incompatible because, if one could overcome these serious methodological problems, one would probably be carrying out research on an atypical sample, using methods that would not be applied in the average mental health service.

Education development

Twelve years ago, the author and a team from the Institute of Psychiatry, London, developed one of the first comprehensive dual diagnosis training programmes in Europe. The central aim of this programme was to provide training in skills in both substance abuse and mental health interventions and provide the student with the necessary range of skills to deal with the various presentations that one finds in patient and community settings. The programme was very much influenced by the earlier development of psychosocial intervention training for nurses, known as the Thorn Programme (Gournay & Birley, 1998). At the same time and shortly after, a number of universities and the Sainsbury Centre for Mental Health developed similar training programmes, and within a few years all parts of the United Kingdom contained very reasonable training courses for health professionals. Obviously, the professional community was proud of this achievement and believed that such training would improve the care given to people with a dual diagnosis. Eventually, a version of the training was developed for testing within a randomised controlled trial (Craig *et al.* 2008). The training consisted of 5 days in the assessment and management of dual diagnosis with subsequent monthly supervision. The interventions used were those supported by the literature as being effective. One of the central elements of the training was therefore motivational interviewing (Swanson *et al.* 1999). The training also focused on training staff in a cognitive behavioural approach to relapse prevention (Irwin *et al.* 1999). The study concerned 79 case managers in 13 London Community Mental Health Teams. Forty of the case managers received training and 39 formed the control group. The effectiveness of the training was measured by the outcomes of the patients with dual diagnosis who were cared for by the respective case managers. The patients were followed up for 18 months. The results showed that training made no difference to drug and alcohol consumption, or days in hospital, although the group of patients allocated to staff who had received the training had significant, though arguably modest, improvement in symptoms and met needs, over and above the control population. While it is true to say that the study was limited by the usual problems associated with research in this area, including high drop-out rates, the results must be disappointing for all concerned, particularly UK policy makers who have for a number of years issued directives relating to increased training for staff and 'mainstreaming' dual diagnosis interventions.

It is obviously essential that the workforce needs to be knowledgeable and skilled enough to meet the needs of patients with a dual diagnosis. However, the unanswered question is, 'What training needs to be delivered?' The results of the studies cited earlier (Johnson *et al.* 2007; Craig *et al.* 2008) suggest that we need to reconsider the balance of the various elements put into training and that, although motivational interviewing and cognitive behavioural approaches to deal with relapse prevention have a reasonable evidence base, we need to consider whether other elements such as medication management training, which also has a good evidence base for people with schizophrenia (Gray *et al.* 2004) need inclusion. The other main issue that needs consideration is whether 5 days of training is long enough to actually improve skills. On the other hand, all public services (not only in the United Kingdom but also elsewhere in the world) face tremendous problems when staff are released for training and one therefore needs to be realistic about the length of training programmes. On the other hand, perhaps we could do more about delivering training in the workplace and, rather than take staff away to classrooms, we might make better use of team meetings to exchange knowledge and skills. Another avenue that might be developed more is that of interactive training using service intranets. It is obvious that much of the material that is delivered in training programmes in classroom settings could be delivered using a computer, and such training could be undertaken by staff at times more convenient to them and the service. This would thus conserve classroom time for skills training sessions and, arguably, maximise the effectiveness of training time away from the service.

Practice

The delivery of services to patients with dual diagnosis has posed a challenge to all mental health services across the world, and how we deliver treatment has been addressed in numerous reviews, articles and chapters (see Proudfoot *et al.* 2003 for an Australian perspective). When one considers practice, one's mind automatically turns to the work of community mental health teams, where much of the problem of dual diagnosis is so evident. This has indeed been the focus of the earlier sections on research and education. However, it might be more helpful to consider practice within a wider context and also consider some further areas, as follows:

- Prevention
- Primary care
- Assessment in mental health and substance abuse services
- Organisation of services
- In-patient care

Prevention

First and foremost, the prevention of the problem should be our primary consideration. It is well known that 50% of current drug dependence can be attributed to pre-existing mental disorders (Kessler *et al.* 2001). Therefore, one might argue that one of the key issues here is early identification of the pre-existing mental disorder and early intervention. One might argue that we should make our early intervention programmes a greater priority and that an integral part of such programmes should be to educate and inform sufferers of mental disorders about the adverse consequences of drug and alcohol use. In a wider sense, the public health perspective is, arguably, the most important area for intervention and we need to ask whether we are doing enough to inform and educate children and adolescents about potential risks of use of drugs and alcohol. We should surely go beyond the 'just say no' approach and ensure that all schools curriculae contain appropriate material on dual diagnosis-related topics.

Primary care

The second area where we need to concentrate practice is in primary care. We know from surveys across the world (e.g. Hickey *et al.* 2001) that many patients with comorbidity present in primary care; these people do not, in the majority, present at mental health or substance abuse services. One therefore might argue that we need to focus our efforts on the education of primary care staff. However, one immediate problem is that such staff will complain that they are already overburdened with 'new' priorities and it is perhaps up to us in the dual diagnosis professional community to persuade primary care staff that dual diagnosis is, indeed, a major priority for intervention and one that cannot be ignored or relegated to an area with 'less important' health priorities.

Assessment in mental health and substance abuse services

The third area of practice on which we need to focus is our assessment processes in substance abuse services and psychiatric services. Across the world, not just in the United Kingdom, it is clear that a divide between substance abuse services and psychiatric services is the single greatest factor in patients with dual diagnosis slipping through the net. In the vast majority of public services across the world, funding for substance abuse and psychiatric services is separate and there is universal recognition that workers in the respective services are, by virtue of their education and training and their practice priorities, often oblivious to issues outside of their domains. While this is understandable, because no one would deny the hard work put in by the average overburdened and underpaid team member, we need to recognise that, now, perhaps the majority of patients attending either substance misuse services or psychiatric services for the first time would meet diagnostic criteria for dual diagnosis. Therefore, perhaps our first training priority should be training all front-line staff in mental health and substance abuse services of robust assessment measures and to obtain agreement about which assessment measures to be used. Such a consensus is currently lacking, and the use of a great variety of methods is unhelpful to say the least.

Organisation of services

The only logical way of addressing the issue of the separation of services which currently exists is at a funding/commissioning level. There must surely be better ways of organising funding so that the considerable divides that currently exist between mental health and substance abuse services and between statutory and voluntary services are, if not abolished, certainly greatly reduced. Many years after dual diagnosis was recognised as a priority for action by various governments across the world, we still have the common situation of the psychiatric patient who is disowned by psychiatric services because of their substance use and the substance-using patient who is disowned by substance abuse services because of their psychiatric problems. Allowing such a situation to continue is to the detriment of not only the individual concerned but also the society more generally.

In-patient care

The other area of potential intervention for patients with dual diagnosis is in the in-patient psychiatric services. A great deal of policy and research has been carried out in community services, but very little emphasis in research and training programmes has been placed in psychiatric in-patient services, where dual diagnosis problems are so clearly expressed. One issue that needs exploration is that of the continuity of care for patients who have been withdrawn from their substances of abuse or alcohol during their in-patient stay and what happens thereafter. Often, in-patient care is a very short-term measure aimed at dealing with the management of risk and it is arguable that we do not use the opportunity to rethink our treatment strategy and, before the patient is discharged, put into place longer term plans. Very often, the dually diagnosed patient will be returned in an improved state, from the point of view of psychiatric symptomatology and, hopefully, in a drug-/alcohol-free state. While the maintenance of psychiatric well-being is often determined by compliance to medication programmes, there is obviously a need to address the issue of recovery from the substance abuse problem. We need to ask whether we are doing enough to put into place active programmes of recovery, of which there are many variants.

The final point to be made about practice is that various elements of practice relating to prevention in schools, widespread screening in general practice, consideration of funding of substance abuse and psychiatric services and the intervention of community mental health teams and in-patient services need to be drawn together, so that our practice is coherent, rather than forming separate strands.

Conclusion

It is by no means novel to say that dual diagnosis is the single greatest priority for mental health and substance abuse services; nor is it novel to say that dual diagnosis is a rising tide. However, it is noteworthy that I can recall using these terms and hearing them from others, in the early and mid-1990s, many years before this book was published. As a community, and I include both those who work in mental health and substance abuse services, we can certainly say that we are all much more cognizant of this problem. Arguably, training programmes have helped us to develop some of the skills needed to deal with the challenges that these patients pose for us. However, we need to ask a simple question: 'What improvements have we made?' While one can cite a range of improvements in practice, education and research, the reality is that, in our society, the problems associated with drug and alcohol use continue to gather momentum. One might argue that while we, in psychiatric and substance abuse services, can make significant contributions, we need to see our efforts in a much wider context and perhaps accept that the solutions to these problems are mainly in political and economic domains, rather than within our control.

References

Barnett J, Werners U, Secher S, *et al.* (2007) Substance use in a population-based clinic sample of people with first episodes of psychosis. *British Journal of Psychiatry* 190: 515–520.

Cleary M, Hunt G, Matherson S, Siegfried N, Walter G (2008) Psychosocial interventions for people with both severe mental illness and substance misuse. *Cochrane Databases: A Systematic Review* (1): ART No. TD0001088.

Craig TKG, Johnson S, McCrone P, *et al.* (2008) Integrated care for co-occurring disorders: psychiatric symptoms, social functioning, and service costs at 18 months. *Psychiatric Services* 59: 276–282.

Frischer M, Collins J, Millson D, Crome I, Croft P (2004) Problems of comorbid psychiatric illness and substance misuse in primary care in England and Wales. *Journal of Epidemiological and Community Health* 58: 1036–1041.

Gournay K, Birley J (1998) The Thorne Programme. *Nursing Times* 94 (49): 54–455.

Gournay K, Sandford T, Johnson S, Thornicroft G (1997) Dual diagnosis of severe mental health problems and substance abuse/dependence: a major priority for mental health nursing. *Journal of Psychiatric and Mental Health Nursing* 4: 89–95.

Gray R, Wykes T, Edmonds M, Leese M, Gournay K (2004) Effect of a medication management training package for nurses on clinical outcomes for patients with schizophrenia: cluster randomised controlled trial. *British Journal of Psychiatry* 185: 157–162.

Hickey I, Koschera A, Davenport T, *et al.* (2001) Comorbidity of common mental disorders and alcohol or other substance misuse in Australian general practice. *Medical Journal of Australia* 175: 31–36.

Irwin J, Bowers C, Dunn M, *et al.* (1999) Efficacy of relapse prevention: a meta-analytic review. *Journal of Consulting and Clinical Psychology* 67: 563–570.

Johnson S, Thornicroft G, Afuwape S, *et al.* (2007) Effects of training community staff in interventions or substance misuse in dual diagnosis patients with psychosis (COMO Study). *British Journal of Psychiatry* 191: 451–452.

Kessler R, Aguilar-Gaxiola S, Andrade L, *et al.* (2001) Mental-substance comorbidities in the ICPE surveys. *Psychiatrica Fennica* 32 (2): 62–79.

Mullaney J, Trippett C (1979) Alcohol dependence and phobias: clinical description and relevance. *British Journal of Psychiatry* 135: 565–573.

Proudfoot H, Teesson M, Briwin E, Gournay K (2003) In: Teesson M, Proudfoot H (eds). *Comorbid Mental Disorders and Substance Abuse Disorders: Epidemiology, Prevention and Treatment*. Canberra: Commonwealth of Australia.

Quitkin F, Rifkin l, Caplan J, Klein D (1972) Phobic anxiety syndrome complicated by drug dependence and addiction: a treatable form of drug abuse. *Archives of General Psychiatry* 27: 159–162.

Swanson A, Pantalon M, Cohen K (1999) Motivational interviewing and treatment adherence among psychiatric and dually diagnosed patients. *Journal of Nervous and Mental Disease* 187: 630–635.

Index

CPSIA information can be obtained at www.ICGtesting.com
Printed in the USA
BVOW09s0850140815

413108BV00002B/1/P